Multidimensional

AROMATHERAPY

Clinical, Practical, and Vibrational Applications

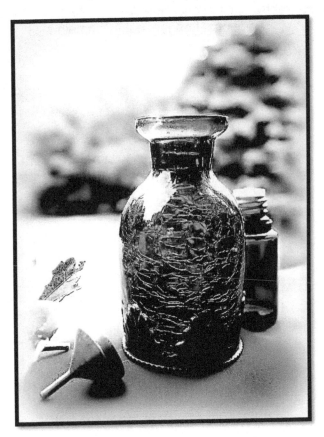

Marlaina Donato, CA, CMT

Ekstasis Multimedia
Blairstown, New Jersey

Multidimensional Aromatherapy/Marlaina Donato
Blairstown, New Jersey: Ekstasis Multimedia, LLC, 2015

ISBN-13: 978-0692418390
ISBN-10: 0692418393

Photography, illustrations, and design: Marlaina Donato
Additional images: public domain

DISCLAIMER

The statements contained herein have not been evaluated by the Food and Drug Administration, and the material presented in this book is not intended to treat, prescribe for, cure, mitigate, or prevent any disease or to replace conventional medical treatments.

Wherever possible, the author has included known contraindications and drug interactions with specific essential oils. Please consult with your medical provider and/or holistic practitioner for possible drug interactions if you are on any medications.

FOR ALL INSPIRED HEALING ARTISTS

WHO SEE MAGIC AND MEDICINE AS A SINGULAR FORCE...

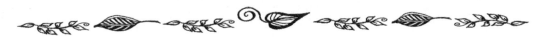

TABLE OF CONTENTS

Part VIII: Vibrational Aromatic Therapy......278

Part IX: Essential Body Care......296

X: Essential Oils in the Treatment Room......312

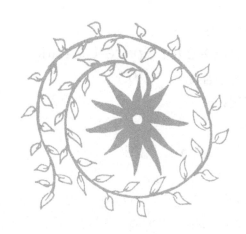

Author's note:

Due to the sometimes trivialized and misunderstood term *aromatherapy*, I have also used the terms *aromatic therapy* and *essential oil therapy* in this work and have chosen to use these terms interchangeably.

This book highlights applications of all three models of essential oil therapy—the British, German, and French. This work does not include clinical ingestion of essential oils found significantly in the French model. As an essential oil therapist I choose to align my practice and approach with *The International Federation of Aromatherapists Code of Ethics* which states:

No aromatherapist shall use essential oils for internal ingestion or internal application nor shall any aromatherapist advocate or promote such use of essential oils **unless** *the practicing aromatherapist has* **medical**, **naturopathic**, **herbalist,** *or similar* **qualifications** *and holds an insurance policy which specifically covers the internal application of essential oils.* (IFA code of ethics. Simply Essential, No. 11 December 1993).

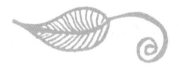

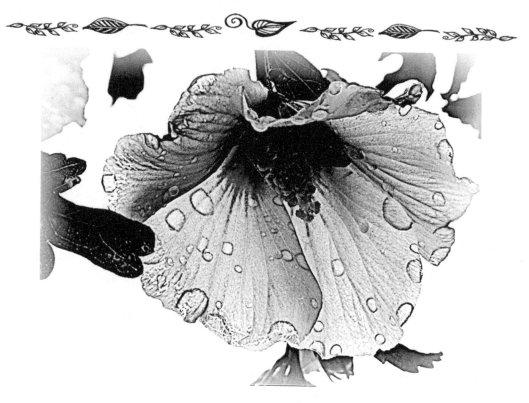

You are invited...

to Multidimensional Aromatherapy,

a crystal-clear approach to a sometimes cryptic practice. Whether you are a beginner, an intermediate student, or a professional in the realm of therapeutic bodywork, Multidimensional Aromatherapy was written with *you* in mind.

Why another book on aromatherapy?

Despite a market already flooded with books on the subject, the average person is prone to believe that aromatherapy equals artificial plug-in air fresheners or celebrity-stamped New Age pleasantries. The more informed individual knows the powerful health benefits of essential oils as well as the blizzard of information (and misinformation), unnecessary details, and polarized material out there geared to either the fad-following novice or the advanced professional. Finally, here is a book that offers beginner's knowledge, intermediate-level approach, and valuable morsels of cutting-

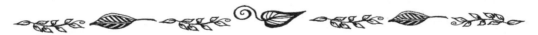

edge information. It also includes twenty years of experience and all of the nuances that come with *living* aromatherapy rather than simply practicing it.

What you won't find in this book...

There are countless books available with detailed information on aspects of aromatic therapy some find interesting and valuable, but if you are like me, you just want to get on with it and get to the meat, cutting away the chaff of information you will probably never use. You may be familiar with the properties of essential oils or blending but still find yourself a bit confused about certain aspects; or you might want to use more aromatherapy applications in your professional practice but need more knowledge about contraindications and medications for client safety. No matter what level you are at in your aromatherapy pursuits, you will not find superfluous minutiae about the intricate workings of steam distillation, excessive history of aromatics and their uses in ancient religious ritual, complex biochemistry of essential oils, chapters on cosmetic perfumery...or any of the interesting but distracting *stuff* that fills the space between covers of too many well-meaning books.

What you will find...

Along the journey of this book, you will find layers of easy-to-access information including:

*square-one basics

*how-to guides without the guesswork

*contraindications and important tips A-Z

*synergistic blending and biochemical overview

*substantial profiles of 100+ essential oils used in aromatherapy including *clinical use / dermal use / inhalation / emotional influence / vibrational influence / chakra correspondence / cosmetic use / tips /caution / notes*

*snippets of cutting-edge clinical findings

*recipes for physical, emotional, and vibrational wellbeing

*inspiring and useful household recipes for chemical-free cleaning

*easy-to-understand explanations of how and why essential oils work in the body, including an outline of critical facts about the nervous system

*vibrational aromatherapy explained from a scientific perspective—*not* trendy New Age lingo

*categorized indexes

*easy-to-create, sumptuous body care products

*essential oil templates for the professional therapeutic bodyworker

and much more.

.

Be informed, be well,

be joyful...and pass it on!

I

ESSENTIAL OIL THERAPY 101

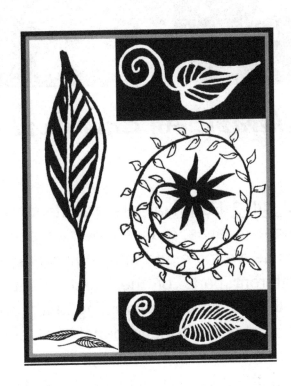

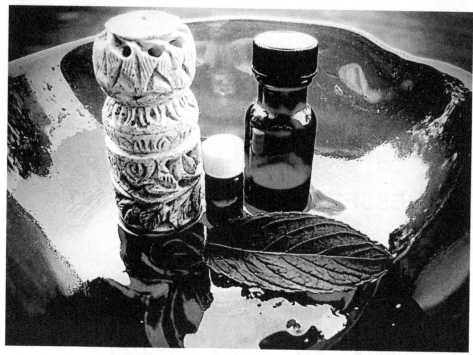

Aromatherapy: An Easy Explanation

What are essential oils? Essential oils are steam-distilled essences of fresh plants, roots, barks, leaves, grasses, berries, seeds, and fruit rinds. A plant's essential oil is its *life force* and *innate immune system that prevents it from disease*. Different parts of the same plant can have different therapeutic effects. Altitude, time of harvesting, and geographic differences of soil all contribute to the therapeutic benefits of essential oils and can vary dramatically from oil to oil. Even though essential oils are commonly believed to be lipids, the oils are actually more akin to water in their undiluted state.

TIP: *In the world of essential oil marketing, as little as only 5% plant material is required for a company to legally state that an essential oil is "100% pure." Please be aware of misleading labels.*

How do they work in the body? When applied to the skin, essential oils are absorbed into the body and the bloodstream within 25 minutes, reaching the deepest cellular levels between 7-12 hours. Essential oils

increase oxygen within the cells, balance the pH factor (acid/alkaline balance essential to life) and can increase the electrical frequency of the body. *Disease and pathogens cannot thrive or survive in an oxygen-abundant environment.* Essential oils can balance hormones, bring harmony to the nervous system, strengthen immunity, kill viruses and bacteria, and offer beneficial effects for many health conditions. When essential oils are inhaled, they affect the limbic part of the brain which governs emotions and the fear response, deep memory banks, and the stress response of fight or flight in the body.

How do essential oils improve the immune system? Essential oils are found in plants and trees and are nature's intrinsic immunity against disease. Once steam-distilled, the concentrated essential oils can boost our own immune response by stimulating the production of white blood cells/antibodies/natural killer cells. Some essential oils are effective if not more effective than pharmaceutical antibiotics without the side effects. Some sources say that it takes *one year* to rebuild beneficial flora in the intestines after *one* round of commonly-prescribed antibiotics. Good bacteria in the bowel comprise the activating force of our immune system, and when this bacterial or flora is compromised, our immunity is weakened. In the conventional world of health, antibiotics are prescribed to fight infection which depletes the intestinal flora that is the very foundation of strong immune response. Multiple rounds of antibiotics keep the immune system weakened indefinitely. We can only imagine what havoc this imposes upon the human body after decades. While antibiotics save lives, they are too often prescribed; collapsed immunity and drug-resistant viruses are the result. *Essential oils, on the other hand, destroy pathogens without killing the vital intestinal flora.* In fact, essential oils have shown to decrease bad intestinal bacteria and increase the beneficial. Essential oils show promising results in the fight against drug-resistant viruses and may be the way of the future.

How do essential oils reduce pain and inflammation? Inflammation is the body's natural attempt to heal what needs to be healed. Due to many factors, this process of inflammation can become chronic, and what began as something beneficial can become problematic. In musculoskeletal

terms, when a muscle is strained or has developed areas of painful tension called *trigger points*, that muscle's state of contraction hinders maximum circulation (blood flow) which prevents adequate cell nutrition; from inadequate circulation and cell nutrition comes a more compromised, painful muscle. Trigger points can deepen and spread. This creates an environment for chronic inflammation which can perpetuate the pain cycle. According to some health care professionals including seasoned chiropractors, this pain cycle of deep trigger points going down five layers of muscle is a major factor in fibromyalgia and myofascial pain syndrome. This explains why some people suddenly develop fibromyalgia after car accidents, falls, and injuries.

On the systemic level, inflammation can result from poor diet, prolonged stress, environmental toxins, and many other factors. Chronic low-level inflammation is now believed to be a major factor in autoimmune diseases, clinical depression, anxiety disorders, heart disease, and even certain types of hair loss. This is where essential oils can play a significantly positive role in our health and wellbeing. Essential oils bring down excessive inflammation and deliver oxygen to the tissues, two critical requirements for multilevel healing. While they cannot be proven to be a panacea, they can certainly improve our quality of life, possibly halt harmful inflammation, and keep our bodies in more of a harmonious state. Essential oils also stimulate endorphins which block pain signals and are invaluable for our everyday injuries, aches and pains, and challenging conditions we humans experience in our physical bodies. Dermal use of essential oils partnered with massage modalities can work wonders for pain reduction, improved circulation, and fewer muscular trigger points.

How do essential oils directly affect the nervous system in relation to anxiety, panic attacks, and depression? The nervous system controls everything in our bodies and is the foundation of life. The functions of the sympathetic branch of the nervous system include the fight or flight response which pumps adrenaline and other stress hormones into our bloodstream so we can either fight or run away from something that threatens our lives. Unfortunately, in our modern times, the sympathetic nervous system doesn't know how to recognize a life-threatening stressor

from a chronic stressor. This means that our fast-paced, ambition-filled, over-scheduled lifestyles kick our sympathetic nervous systems into overdrive. Adrenalin and cortisol are produced so we can handle a crisis, but these stress hormones secreted from the adrenals are not designed to keep pumping out. The brain continues to signal the adrenals to secrete these stress hormones, and these poor, tiny glands don't get a rest when our bodies constantly respond to stimuli. Excessive cortisol and adrenaline can lead to obesity, exhaustion, heart disease, chronic anxiety, and chronic inflammation, just to name a few.

On the other hand, the *parasympathetic* branch of the nervous system is responsible for the body's "rest and digest" mode. Anything pleasurable including being in nature or getting a massage signals the parasympathetic nervous system to kick in, and when it does, the fight or flight response finally turns off. Not all of us can schedule regular massage sessions and vacations into our lives, and this is where regular use of essential oils can spare our bodies from the ravages of the chronic stress response.

Essential oils, especially when inhaled, affect the release of neurotransmitters, chemical messengers in the body that play a vital role in the nervous system. Neurotransmitters like serotonin and dopamine (to name only two) are the chemical messengers in the body that shape our moods and behaviors. Chronic stress, poor diet, hormone imbalances, traumatic events, overwork, emotional heartache, substance abuse, excessive alcohol and coffee consumption, and too little sleep can alter our neurotransmitter production, thus putting us onto a merry-go-round of added stress. Eating disorders, clinical depression, Obsessive Compulsive Disorder (OCD), panic attacks, phobias, and addictive tendencies can manifest from neurotransmitter imbalances and can be a never-ending loop of physiological and psychological triggers. Inhaling essential oils such as lavender, cacao, rose, and sweet orange stimulates neurotransmitter production within seconds. Applying them to the body to be absorbed into the skin also nourishes the nervous system.

Essential oils also have a profound effect on brain waves. Oils such as Roman chamomile, bergamot, lavender, and melissa induce alpha waves,

the rhythm of the brain associated with dreams and the level that is most conducive for using positive affirmations. Jasmine, rose, and neroli induce theta waves, the rhythm of sleep. (For more on the nervous system, neurotransmitters, and emotional wellbeing, see page 222)

Types of Aromatherapy Application

Practical Aromatherapy is the application of essential oils in everyday living. Practical uses of oils can include cleaning/disinfecting, First-Aid, gardening, air-freshening, pet health, and cooking (only high-quality essential oils can be ingested. Know your sources and apply only after extensive knowledge is gained in this area.)

Clinical Aromatherapy is the application of high-quality essential oils for physical, emotional, and mental well-being. Methods of application can include *dermal* (through the skin via diluted blends or neat through the soles of the feet), *diffusion* (releasing particles into the air), *inhalation*, and *ingestion* (found in the French model of aromatherapy under strict supervision by a medical physician or a certified clinical aromatherapist with a medical or herbal background.) Clinical aromatherapy can be highly beneficial for countless health concerns including serious infections, PMS, menopause, insomnia, unstable blood sugar and blood pressure, pain, endocrine balance, adrenal exhaustion, panic/anxiety, cystic breasts, pH balance, acute and chronic stress, and much more.

FAST FACT: *In France, only medical doctors can administer essential oils.*
Tip: Advanced clinical aromatherapy is often called Medical Aromatherapy.

Cosmetic Aromatherapy is the application of essential oils in skin health and beauty routines. Cosmetic aromatherapy can include skin care, deodorants, bath products, natural or holistic perfumery, and hydrosols.

FAST FACT: *In the cosmetic industry, a single lab-created fragrance can have up to 500 artificial chemicals in its composition. Many health food store brands of cosmetics, soaps, and bath products claim to be "organic" or "all natural" when in reality the fragrance in the product is synthetic and made from petroleum-based chemicals. Unless a product label states "natural fragrance" and/or lists essential oils including Latin botanical names, it is most likely artificial. Sometimes a label will list both essential oils by name and also have a listing for "perfume" or "fragrance" which indicates artificial and natural ingredients.*

Vibrational Aromatherapy is the application of essential oils that directly affects the vibrational frequency of the body which also includes the subtle realms of emotional and spiritual wellbeing. Vibrational aromatherapy can also be applied to get to the energetic or root cause of some physical and/or emotional health complaints. Much like all living beings, each essential oil possesses frequency. Essential oil frequency is measured by megahertz (MHz). It is believed that high-vibrational oils can raise the frequency of an individual or environment and thus improve wellbeing. When used synergistically, essential oils can also stimulate the pituitary and pineal glands which some believe to play a role in spiritual, mystical, and/or psychic experience. Application can be employed with other techniques including energy work and Reiki, hands-on-healing, prayer, and other energetic modalities. Vibrational aromatic therapy can be highly beneficial for healing deep emotional trauma and past abuse. Some children and adults with ADD/ADHD may see improvement using vibrational applications. (For a scientific perspective and overview of the energetic network, see page 279.)

FAST FACT: *Essential oils range in frequency from 53 MHz (basil) to 320 MHz (rose), but individual people, emotions, electrical appliances, and even atmospheric pressure can increase or decrease their frequencies.* **Tip:** An essential oil's frequency can be raised if combined with another essential oil that is higher in frequency. Rose, the highest of frequencies, is known to raise the frequency of all essential oils that may be combined with it and makes a valuable addition to any blend.

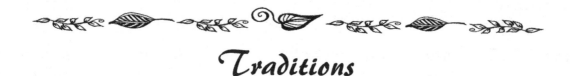

Traditions

The British Model: This tradition of aromatic therapy focuses on dilution of essential oils and dermal application with or without massage modalities.

The French Model: This tradition of aromatic therapy focuses on medical aromatherapy, ingestion of essential oils and dermal application using undiluted essential oils. Undiluted dermal application includes applying essential oils to the soles of the feet where the pores are largest in the body, therefore ensuring quicker delivery into the bloodstream. Some practitioners advocate undiluted application of essential oils on other parts of the body other than the soles of the feet. Due to the fact that we are all individual—especially regarding body chemistry and skin sensitivity—and based upon my experiences with clients, this book only discusses neat application to the soles of the feet.

The German Model: This tradition of aromatic therapy significantly highlights inhalation methods and their effect on the brain, especially functions of the hypothalamus (which governs hormonal activity in the entire body) and limbic system (which controls fear, anxiety, and other emotional responses.)

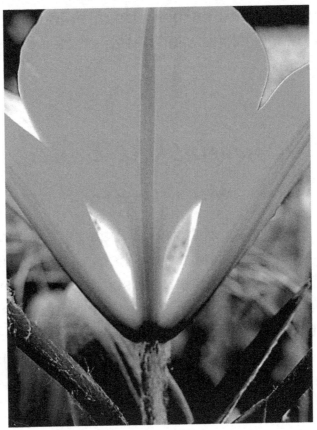

Aromatic History in a Nutshell

FAST FACTS:

The use of aromatic plants is a global common ground throughout the ancient world. Evidence in various cultures suggests that the use of aromatics dates back to 4,000 B.C. or even earlier. Some uses included mummification, ritual and ceremonial use, beauty regimens, cooking, and medicine.

Stream distillation is attributed to the Persians; the renowned 11th century physician Avicenna invented the refrigerated coil in the distillation process. He wrote an entire book on the medicinal properties of the rose which was also the first plant he steam distilled successfully.

French biochemist René-Maurice Gattefossé was the first to use the term "aromatherapy" in the 1920s. He attributed lavender essential oil to his profound recovery from gas gangrene.

French Army physician and surgeon Jean Valnet used essential oils on wounded soldiers during World War II with profound results, especially in treatment of gangrene.

Essential Oil Basics

What to Look For

Essential oils are composed of complex natural chemical structures, and synthetic oils can never duplicate their therapeutic value. Using synthetic oils or compromised (adulterated) essential oils not only nets *zero therapeutic benefits* but increases health risks including skin rash, allergies, and putting extra burden on the lungs, kidneys, and liver. Please bear this in mind if you are tempted to purchase inexpensive oils that you think smell like the "real thing." There is no such thing as a $5 bottle of undiluted rose oil or lavender oil that is purple. Synthetics possess zero frequency.

Except for citrus, there are no true *essential oils* of fruits. If you see an "essential oil" of *strawberry, raspberry, peach, apple, melon*, etc., it is synthetic, even if it includes "natural" on the label. Flower "oils" such as *violet* (not to be confused with violet leaf), *wisteria*, and *honeysuckle* are chemically-based and contain little if any plant essentials. *French vanilla* is another "oil" that does not exist in therapeutic essential oils. Most commercial products in your local supermarket with "aromatherapy" or "lavender" on the label <u>do not contain any essential oils</u>; this includes laundry detergents, fabric softeners, dish soaps, baby shampoo, lotions, bar soap, hand soap, deodorants/antiperspirant, body fragrances, facial cleansers and masks, skin products, candles, and air fresheners. To be sure the product of choice is authentic, make sure the list of ingredients includes the Latin botanical plant names and be aware of false advertising. *Rule of thumb:* Oils labeled as "fragrance oil" are *not* essential oils, and not all brands of *essential* oils are equal in therapeutic value or company integrity. Many are suitable for cosmetic use such as soap-making and perfumery but are not recommended for clinical application.

Appearance: True therapeutic essential oils are usually colorless, amber, golden, or pale green in color. There are naturally occurring blue essential oils such as German chamomile, blue cypress, blue tansy, and blue yarrow. Aside from this unique group, avoid any products that have intense colors as well as any oils sold in *clear* bottles. **Tip:** A pure essential oil will not leave a stain on paper or tissue. If an essential oil leaves a stain, it is most likely "cut" with unwanted additives. Diluted essential oils, on the other hand, will leave a stain due to the carrier oil, which is expected. Diluted essential oils are clearly labeled.

Identification: *Always be sure* that the labels on your chosen essential oils include their botanical Latin identification. **e.g.** lavender (*Lavandula angustifolia*). Botanical names ensure accuracy when identifying essential oils, certain species, and come in handy when purchasing an essential oil that has a name similar to that of another. **e.g.** bay and bay Laurel or ravensara and ravintsara.

Shelf life: Essential oils have varying shelf life. Oils extracted from roots, barks, spices, and heartwood last the longest and can even improve with age. Those such as citrus have the shortest shelf life and should be used within six months after opening for optimum results. All essential oils must be kept away from direct sunlight, artificial light, heat, and electrical sources to maximize their freshness and therapeutic frequency. **Tip:** citrus oils used in dermal blends or household cleaning sprays can be preserved quite effectively if combined with essential oils such as clove.

Therapeutic concentration: Even so-called "reputable" essential oil companies can use undesirable solvents in their extraction process or cut costs by sneaking in other oils to "stretch" the scent of a particular oil. **e.g.** jasmine absolute stretched with ylang ylang essential oil or rose absolute stretched with rose geranium. The most commonly adulterated essential oils are jasmine, sandalwood, frankincense, and rose. See Resources for reputable suppliers.

True Aroma: Essential oils are highly concentrated and often are mis-

leading at first whiff from the bottle. Only dilution or exposure on the skin for a few minutes can reveal the true scent.

Where to Purchase: Essential oil companies vary in terms of sources, integrity, and process of essential oils. Some, not all, health food store brands are acceptable for clinical use, but there are better, high-quality options that should be considered. Health food store brands often produce only the most commonly used essential oils; luckily, today there are many options to choose from. Please see Resources for companies that carry a broad range of essential oils.

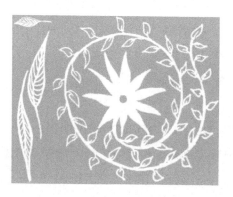

Methods of Application

DERMAL METHOD
(Through the Skin)

1. <u>Diluted in a carrier or base oil</u>

This method is widely used for massage or for distributing the benefits of essential oils over large areas of the body. Especially useful for muscle pain and injury, and balancing the nervous system.

Most useful for: strains, sprains, fibromyalgia, osteoarthritis, hormonal balance; also used for cosmetic applications.

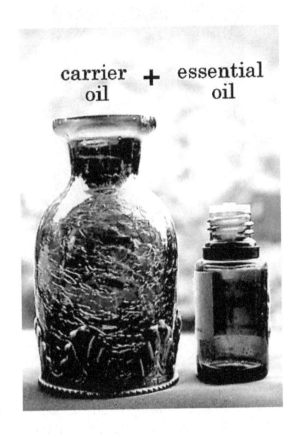

carrier + essential
oil   oil

How: Add essential oils to any carrier or base oil and apply to the body. Examples of carrier/base oils: grapeseed, jojoba, safflower, light olive, liquefied coconut, and almond. See page 45 for details.

2. <u>Applied Undiluted </u>(called neat)

Due to individual skin sensitivity, neat application of essential oils is recommended to the soles of the feet. Pores of the foot sole are the largest in the body, therefore ideal for fast delivery of essential oils into the bloodstream.

Most useful for: hormonal balance, optimal oxygen delivery to tissues and organs, and acute conditions such as cold, influenza, and bacterial and viral infection. Excellent for maintaining strong immunity, especially through the winter months

How: Apply oils to the soft part of the foot sole between the ball of the foot and the heel.

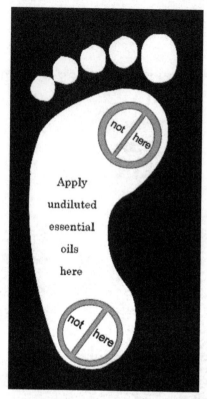

In the British Model of essential oil therapy, due to concentration of essential oils and individual sensitivity, it is advised to not apply essential oils _neat_—except for lavender and a couple of other specified essential oils—to any other part of the body.

Bath and Footbath

Involves adding essential oils to Epsom salts, sea salt, or a similar agent and adding the salts to bath water or a foot soak.

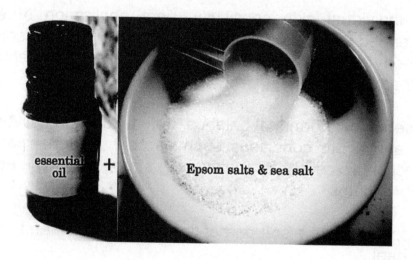

Most useful for: calming the nervous system, boosting immunity, and receiving the benefits of inhalation along with absorption of essential oils through the skin.

How: Add essential oil(s) to a base of Epsom salts and/or sea salt (See page 248 for details and recipes.)

Spray Misters

Essential oils are added to distilled water or rose water and sprayed on the body for absorption.

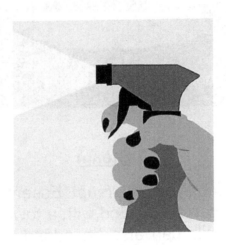

Most useful for: skin health, cosmetic use of fragrance/perfume, and cooling the body during summer months.

How: Add essential oil(s) to a spray bottle filled ¾ with distilled water (See page 302 for fragrant body spritzers.)

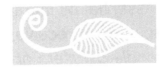

INHALATION METHOD

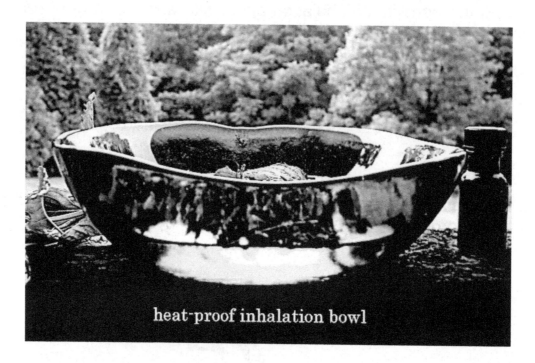

heat-proof inhalation bowl

1. <u>Steam</u>

This method can be employed via *steam*. Essential oils are dropped into a bowl of hot water and can be inhaled with a towel over the head to form a steam tent. Essential oils can also be added to the sides of the tub or shower and released into the air as the water runs hot. Oils can be also dropped onto a wet wash cloth in a steam room or dry sauna.

most useful for: sinus congestion/pain/pressure, colds, uplifting mood (See page 243 for details and recipes.)

2. <u>Diffusion</u>

This inhalation method is applied by using a *nebulizer* or *ultrasonic diffuser* to release fine particles of essential oil into the air to kill bacteria, airborne viruses, and molds. It is also used to receive optimum benefit from inhaling essential oils. **Tip**: *Avoid candle diffusers or any diffuser that uses heat or a candle. These are not true essential oil diffusers and have little, if any, therapeutic effect. Heat destroys all vital properties of essential oils. Candle diffusers are not taken seriously by professionals who truly want*

the maximum therapeutic benefits of aromatic oils. Plug-in and reed "diffusers" for home and the car can affect mood and scent the immediate area but *do not* destroy bacteria or viruses or boost the immune system.

Most useful for: disinfecting the air of sick rooms and preventing infectious agents from spreading from person to person. Also valuable to uplift mood, calm anxiety, or induce sleep. It is lovely way to scent your home or provide a healthy environment for clients in professional settings. Diffusers and nebulizers vary in price, and higher-end models are recommended to avoid malfunction and to guarantee the fullest potential of the device.

3. <u>Handkerchief or Aroma Locket</u>

The is the easiest method of inhalation anytime, anywhere. A few drops will last for hours (sometimes days, depending upon which oils are used) and can be kept in a plastic bag for freshness. Aromatic necklaces/lockets are also available for the same purpose. This method affects the brain/limbic system and is highly effective for mood elevation and control of anxiety *but it does not kill viruses and bacteria.*

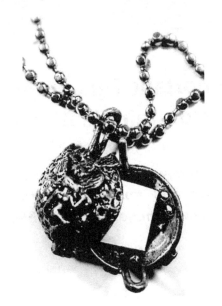

Most useful for: taking essential oils with you wherever you go-especially to the workplace where it is not practical to use essential oils

from the bottle. Ideal for people who use essential oils to control anxiety or who simply want an alternative to wearing perfume.

How: add a drop or two of essential oil on a tissue; fold over once or twice to avoid oils being in direct contact with the skin or eyes. Inhale a few times a day, no longer than 5-10 minutes at a time. If using an aroma locket, add a few drops to a diffuser pad, put it inside the locket, and wear around the neck, or keep in a pocket to use whenever desired. **Tip:** wearing an aroma locket close to the skin will be gently warmed by body heat, enhancing and bringing out the scent of the oils.

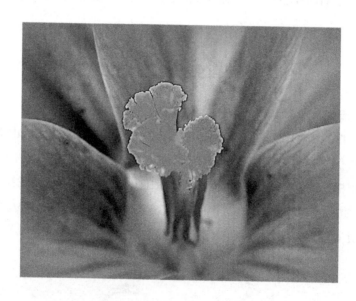

Very Important Tips, Information, and Contraindications A-Z

<u>**Author's Note:**</u> *This is an overview of important information that can be found in one place; contraindications and tips specific to each essential oil profile (Section II) have also been added whenever applicable.*

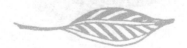

<u>**Absorption:**</u> For maximum absorption into the body, essential oils should remain on the skin for four-seven hours; be sure to allow the oils to

penetrate the tissues, and do not bathe *after* applying them. The easiest way to do this is to apply essential oils in the morning after showering or before bed. To gain the best results possible from using essential oils dermally, do not blend essential oils with *scented* body lotion and body lotion found in most supermarkets that are produced by large, recognizable brands; these most often contain chemicals that can interfere with treatments and produce unwanted effects such as skin rashes.

Addiction recovery: As a rule of thumb, half the recommended amount of essential oils is best for anyone dealing with an active addiction or newly recovering, for the liver is in process of recuperating, and a little essential oil therapy goes a long way without risk of stressing an already burdened organ.

Alcohol: See **Intoxication**

Anxiety: Individuals prone to anxiety, panic attacks, and nervousness should avoid stimulating essential oils such as coffee, nutmeg, and sometimes ginger essential oil. Discontinue use if anxiety is worsened. Ginger, both as a supplement and essential oil, *may decrease available serotonin* in the body which can interfere with pharmaceutical antidepressants.

Asthma: While essential oil application can ease an asthmatic attack, *never* use essential oils directly near the face of those with asthmatic conditions. Always apply to the soles of the feet. In general, peppermint and any menthol-containing essential oils (camphor, spearmint, eucalyptus, white thyme, cajeput, and sage) should be avoided in all cases of asthma as menthol can trigger asthma attacks in some individuals. If it is certain that menthol can be tolerated without problems, use such oils with caution and in small amounts.

Blood sugar: *Sweet fennel, coriander, cedar, clary sage, goldenseal, goldenrod, geranium, dill, Roman chamomile, myrrh,* and *ylang ylang* may help the pancreas secrete insulin, and if applied to the skin or soles of the

feet, should be used with caution; required dose for insulin or medication could be altered due to the blood sugar-lowering effects of these essential oils. *Except for inhalation*, these oils should be also used in small amounts or avoided by anyone with reactive/non-diabetic hypoglycemia (low blood sugar). *Angelica* essential oil should also be avoided by diabetics.

Botanical names: There are essential oils that have similar names but are very different from each other and not related. Latin botanical names on labels help clarify what is actually in the bottle and differentiate between species. Two oils that might seem similar or two oils that share some of the same actions often have distinctly different properties or have different contraindications.

Cancer: Though some essential oils have proven to be allies in fighting certain cancers, there are some oils that are contraindicated if someone has or has had estrogen-dependent cancer and prostate cancer. Certain sources recommend that some essential oils be avoided if you have or have had prostate cancer, especially *bay* (Pimenta racemosa). If you have or had estrogen-dependent cancer, including that of the breast, it is recommended that you avoid *anise, star anise, clary sage*, and *sweet fennel* essential oils. Oils to *avoid if you've had any type of cancer* include: *bay* (Pimenta racemosa) and *clary sage*. See **Chemotherapy and Radiation Therapy.**

Caustic oils: Due to chemical concentration, cinnamon, clove, thyme, and oregano oils should never be used on the skin except for highly diluted applications *or on the soles of the feet.*

Chemical Compounds: In clinical terms, essential oils are grouped by their dominant chemical compounds including **alcohols** (a.k.a. monoterpenes), **phenols, esters, aldehydes, ketones** (also spelled as cetons), **ethers**, and **sesquiterpenes**. Those highest in phenols such as oregano and clove can be powerful and highly irritating to the skin if used improperly while oils such as lavender with a high ester content are considered safest on the skin. Essential oils high in sesquiterpenes such as

frankincense and sandalwood oxygenate the brain and are especially calming to the nervous system. Essential oil biochemistry is the focus of advanced/medical aromatherapy for both synergy and safety. (See page 50 for an overview of essential oil chemistry groups and their properties in relation to synergy.)

Chemotherapy and Radiation Therapy: Certain essential oils enhance the effectiveness of anti-nausea drugs given during and after chemotherapy. Essential oils recommended to lessen nausea from cancer treatments include cardamom, German chamomile, and ginger. See the profiles of these individual oils for more information. Niaoli essential oil can be used to diminish harmful effects of radiation therapy. Ravintsara essential oil used dermally will also lessen the side effects of the drug Interferon.

Costly oils: Costly essential oils such as rose, jasmine, Roman and German chamomile, neroli, sandalwood, angelica root, melissa (lemon balm), and carrot seed are also sold in diluted form and are very affordable. Keep this in mind when you read about a full-strength essential oil that is beyond your budget. The therapeutic value is not compromised by dilution, and the scent is most often lovelier than its concentrated form.

Children: Always keep essential oils out of reach of children. When applying essential oils to children, it is recommended to use 1/10 of the recommended amount for adults. (See page 46 for ratio according to children's age groups.) **Do not** use *peppermint* essential oil on a child or infant; however, diffusion via nebulizer is safe when the child is not asthmatic. Do not use *eucalyptus* or *cajeput* on a young child or infant, for menthol is too concentrated and can be toxic. *Cinnamon bark* essential oil should not be used on children, nor should it be diffused via nebulizer when children are present. There are many oils that are safe and recommended for children such as lavender, Roman and German chamomile, melissa (lemon balm), and others. (See page 70 for a list of essential oils suitable and safe for children and babies.)

Dilution: Except for *lavender, tea tree, helichrysum*, and small applications of *rosewood* essential oil, it is recommended that *all essential oils be diluted in a carrier oil or lotion before dermal application.* **However**, essential oils can be used *undiluted* on the soles of the feet where the pores are the largest in the body, thus enabling immediate absorption. This application usually poses no risk of rash or unpleasant effects due to the less-sensitive, tougher skin. Despite the gentleness of lavender, tea tree, and helichrysum essential oils, some individuals are sensitive. Dilute if need be. (See page 44 for types of carrier oils, blending, and ratio recommendations.)

Dilution for Baths: Essential oils intended for bath use should always be stirred into Epsom salts or sea salt, unscented shower gel, or shampoo so they can dissolve evenly in the water. If not distributed this way, essential oils tend to float on the surface of the water and can cause skin irritation.

Epilepsy/Seizure Disorders: *Rosemary, sweet fennel, tarragon, dill, anise seed, star anise, wintergreen, sweet birch,* and *carrot seed/root,* and *hyssop* essential oils should be avoided by anyone prone to seizures or epilepsy. Both dermal use *and* inhalation are not recommended.

Fevers: Some oils such as peppermint are recommended to help bring down adult fevers while others are strongly contraindicated. Essential oils to avoid with fever are the oils considered "hot" such as *cinnamon bark* and *ginger. Peppermint is contraindicated for children's fever; use lavender instead.* As a rule of thumb, fevers are natural and part of the body's defense against bacteria and viruses. Fevers are only dangerous when they reach high temperatures, and in such cases, medical treatment should be sought.

First-Aid: In case of accidental swallowing of essential oils, call the Poison Control Center immediately. If essential oils should get into your eyes, do not flush with water; flush the eye with light vegetable oil until discomfort subsides. For severe cases of essential oils getting into the eyes, seek immediate medical treatment. In my personal experience, a warm flush of

water *after thoroughly treating with vegetable oil* works best. Please be aware of having oils on your fingers and then rubbing your face or eyes, especially lemongrass and anything with menthol including *peppermint, spearmint,* and *eucalyptus.*

Flammability: Essential oils are flammable. Keep away from fire/open flames.

Frequency of Use: Along with food what we ingest and which cosmetics we put on our skin, the liver metabolizes essential oils. Due to the concentration of essential oils, it is wise to use them dermally at a pace that the liver can metabolize in order to receive optimum results. Less is more.

Furniture: Avoid applying or spilling undiluted essential oils directly on furniture, for essential oils can harm fine wood finishes.

Heart Rhythm Disorders: Individuals with heart rhythm disorders should avoid direct inhalation and dermal use of *coffee* and *nutmeg* essential oil to avoid possible adverse reactions.

Hemophilia: Anyone with hemophilia should not **dermally** use *bay, clove bud, cinnamon leaf, cinnamon bark, bay laurel, wintergreen, oregano, sweet birch, lemongrass, ginger, anise seed, star anise, carrot seed/root, Roman and German chamomile, yarrow, marjoram, all citrus (lemon, sweet orange, mandarin, tangerine, bergamot), melissa (lemon balm), clary sage,* and *cassia* essential oils.

High blood pressure: *Peppermint, eucalyptus, pine, cypress, ginger, rosemary, juniper berry, thyme, sage,* and *Texas cedar* essential oils have long been assumed to raise blood pressure, and this information has been published and re-published for decades despite convincing evidence. In his 2010 in-depth article about essential oils and hypertension, renowned aromatherapist and author Robert Tisserand stated that these oils *should be taken off the advisory list* for high blood pressure; in fact, there are studies that show some of these oils actually lower blood pressure- quite

the opposite of what we've been told. Tisserand also stated that *inhaling grapefruit, lemon, caraway, black pepper, sweet fennel*, or *tarragon* essential oil for 10 minutes has been shown to increase blood pressure *slightly* for a *brief* time.

Homeopathic interaction: Peppermint essential oil along with other menthol-containing oils such as spearmint and eucalyptus may neutralize homeopathic remedies. Avoid these oils 2 hours before and after employing homeopathic remedies.

Hyperthyroidism: Individuals with *hyper*thyroidism should avoid *green myrtle* essential oil for it has shown to increase thyroid hormone.

Hypothyroidism: Individuals with *hypo*thyroidism should not use sweet fennel of *melissa* (lemon balm) essential oil for long periods, for the herb itself is contraindicated for low thyroid function.

Immunity: Rotating the use of immune-boosting essential oils is necessary to prevent the body from getting used to their specific actions and chemistry. For example, if tea tree oil or lavender is used daily, the body will become immune, and the effects of the oils will be greatly diminished, if not cancelled out. **Tip:** To avoid this, rotate with other oils with similar properties. For example, use tea tree oil combined with lavender for a week and then switch to another appropriate combination such as organic lemon and clove.

Ingestion: Ingestion of essential oils, though championed by many sources within the field of essential oil practice, is not for everyone. Essential oils are highly concentrated substances, *higher than they are found in their natural state*, and the liver often cannot metabolize this concentration of chemical compounds quickly enough and can prove to cause negative side effects, especially if toxins in the body cannot be flushed out at a timely pace. Despite many claims, ingestion of essential oils can prove to be dangerous without proper guidance. There are companies, representatives, and consultants who will beg to differ with these statements. There are

countless people who ingest essential oils without concrete knowledge, and for many, it can be beneficial; however, every **body** is different and reacts differently in any given circumstance. In today's world of widespread prescribed drugs, interactions *are more likely than any previous decade*. As a professional essential oil practitioner, I suggest to you, the reader, to remain on the side of caution, retain logic, and healthy skepticism. In France, only medical doctors can administer essential oils. I believe wholeheartedly that there is a reason for this. It is recommended that ingestion of essential oils be advised and guided by a *certified clinical* aromatherapist with an appropriate and documented medical, herbal, or naturopathic background.

Inhalation: Small intervals of time are recommended for inhalation of essential oils. Some individuals are more sensitive to essential oils, especially to pungent aromas such as basil, ylang ylang, and jasmine. If headache or other unpleasant symptoms result, simply inhale for shorter periods of time or substitute with milder scents.

Intoxication: Avoid *clary sage* essential oil when drinking or taking certain medications that affect dopamine production, for it can increase neurotransmitter levels in the brain, thus intensifying the effects of alcohol and certain medications. *Bay* (Pimenta racemosa) and *star anise* (Illicium verum) are also oils to avoid, especially by individuals addicted to alcohol. These same precautions are recommended for anyone using recreational drugs.

Kidney Disease: Individuals with kidney disease or a history of kidney disease should avoid concentrated *dermal use* of *juniper berry* essential oil. If kidney disease or compromised kidney function is evident, *dermal use* of *lemon* essential oil should also be avoided.

Lavender, Myrrh, and Ginger Essential Oils: According to some medical aromatherapists, adding a bit of lavender essential oil to blends or combinations will assure quicker and more reliable delivery of beneficial

properties of the other oils. Myrrh and ginger essential oils also enhance the actions of any essential oils combined with them.

Liver Disease: Individuals with liver disease should not use *star anise* or *anise seed* essential oils. It is also recommended that individuals with liver disease approach dermal applications of essential oils with these guidelines: *properly dilute, double dilute, and give plenty of time between applications* in order for the liver to have time to process essential oils without burdening an already compromised organ.

Long-term use: Oils such as rosemary, sweet birch, and wintergreen contain powerful chemical components that can accumulate in the body and can be harmful if used consistently over time. To be on the safe side, do not use these oils daily or habitually in *dermal* applications.

Low blood pressure: Lavender and lemon essential oils can lower, as well as stabilize, blood pressure; however, caution is recommended in severe cases of hypotension (low blood pressure.)

Massage: Using essential oils during a bodywork session will lessen or prevent post-massage soreness. Most therapists are glad to incorporate any oils you'd like to use during the session. The best ones to choose from are: *balsam fir, pine needle, spearmint, or peppermint.* Highly recommended for anyone with fibromyalgia or receiving deep tissue work.

Medication contraindications: Those allergic or sensitive to **aspirin** should not use *sweet birch* or *wintergreen* essential oil. *Ginger* and *lemongrass* essential oils should be avoided by those on certain medications including **blood thinners**. Those who are cautioned to avoid the intake of **ginger** in the diet due to medication contraindications should also avoid *dermal use and inhalation* of ginger essential oil. Individuals on blood thinners should also avoid or use the following oils with extreme caution: *bay, clove bud, cinnamon leaf, cinnamon bark, bay laurel, wintergreen, oregano, sweet birch, anise seed, star anise, carrot seed/root, Roman and German chamomile, yarrow, marjoram, all citrus including lemon, sweet orange, mandarin, tangerine, bergamot, melissa (lemon*

balm), *clary sage*, and *cassia* essential oils. Anyone using **paracetamol** should not use *star anise* essential oil (Illicium verum). *Ginger*, both as a supplement and essential oil, may decrease available serotonin which can interfere with both pharmaceutical and supplemental **antidepressants**. Individuals using pharmaceutical and supplemental antidepressants should be cautious when using mood-enhancing essential oils such as *ginger, clary sage, anise, star anise, lavender, all citrus, ylang ylang, neroli*, and *rose*, for these oils may alter the required dose of needed medication. Check with your doctor or pharmacist. See **Intoxication** for further info on medications and certain oils.

Mucus membranes: Avoid direct contact with eyes, nose, mouth, and the genital area; essential oils are extremely concentrated.

Pesticides: Citrus essential oils are cold-pressed from fruit rinds. To avoid considerable amounts of pesticides, use only *organic citrus* essential oils for dermal application. **Tip:** Some companies are now offering steam-distilled citrus essential oils which contain far less pesticide residue, namely lime essential oil.

Pets: Pets, particularly cats and dogs, are highly sensitive to essential oils. It is recommended that undiluted oils do not come in contact with your pet except for minimal amounts added to bath water (for dogs.) **Tip:** some essential oils such as peppermint, eucalyptus, tea tree, and lavender are excellent flea repellants, deodorizers, and skin-soothers that can be added to bath water. **Caution:** according to some sources, lavender, tea tree, and peppermint essential oils may be harmful to cats, for their livers process essential oils differently, even when oils are inhaled.

Photosensitivity: *All citrus* essential oils (**e.g.** lemon, mandarin, tangerine, orange, grapefruit, lime, palmarosa, and bergamot), *angelica, lovage, lemongrass, cumin, lemon verbena, tagetes*, and sometimes *ginger* and *spruce* oils can cause skin and sun sensitivity. As a rule of thumb, when using these oils in dermal applications, skin should not be exposed to direct sunlight or tanning beds for 24-48 hours after application.

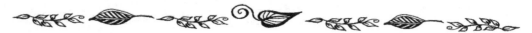

Pregnancy and Breastfeeding: Extreme caution should be used during pregnancy. Some schools of thought believe oils should be avoided completely while others believe a few are beneficial and safe. Diluted rose and mandarin essential oils are considered safe during pregnancy, and frankincense is said to ease the process of labor. Consult a certified, seasoned clinical aromatherapist before using any oils during pregnancy or breastfeeding.

Sage Essential Oil: According to many sources, the only sage oil considered safe for *dermal* application is clary sage.

Scent preferences: As a rule of thumb, go with what scents appeal to individual tastes at the time, for the body has a way of telling us what it needs by what we are drawn to.

Scented Lotions: Essential oils should not be blended with *scented* lotions, creams, or carrier oils; the carrier or base oil must be pure and unscented as possible to retain the integrity of the essential oils. Essential oils mixed with synthetic chemical ingredients can cause unwanted skin reactions and compromise therapeutic potency of the oils.

Storage: Always store essential oils and carrier oils in a cool place out of direct sunlight. Avoid heat sources including heat vents, fire places, and kitchen stoves. Keep away from televisions, computers, cell phones and microwaves, for all of these will compromise the therapeutic value and lower the energetic frequency of essential oils.

Synergy: Synergistic blending of essential oils is the hallmark of a well-intentioned aromatherapist or bodyworker. Single essential oils have significant properties, but combining oils for specific concerns can help speed healing, induce wellbeing, and ease a client through life changes. Synergy is a biochemical and intuitive art—a holistic science that can take years of experienced study and practice, but specially-blended formulas for specific conditions can be easy to prepare with a few basic guidelines. <u>Tip:</u> "Synergistic to" does not mean "smells nice when blended with."

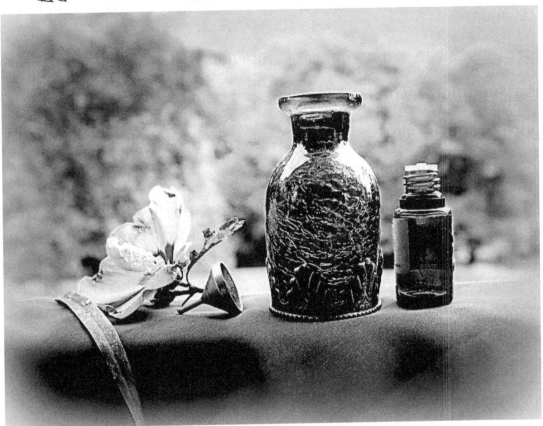

Common Useful Definitions

Absolute: essential oil extracted through a process involving alcohol e.g. jasmine, rose, and other specific florals

Analgesic: pain blocking e.g. peppermint, lavender, eucalyptus, clove

Anticatarrhal: lessens inflammation of the mucus membranes e.g. frankincense, eucalyptus

Anticoagulant: minimizes clotting of the blood e.g. ginger, lemongrass

Antidepressant: lessens symptoms of depression by raising or balancing neurotransmitters that affect mood e.g. lavender, basil, clary sage

Antifungal: lessens or prevents the overgrowth of fungus e.g. tea tree oil, lavender, rosewood

Antihistamine: lessens the effects of histamine during an allergic reaction

e.g. lavender

Antiseptic: inhibits microorganisms from flourishing e.g. all essential oils

Antispasmodic: lessens spasms e.g. peppermint

Antiviral: combats viruses

Base oil see **Carrier Oil**

Chakra: from Eastern philosophy; etheric energy centers within the physical body and energy field of an individual that correspond to specific organs and regions. It is commonly believed that there are seven chakras. According to many schools of thought and those in the healing arts, the number of chakras varies and is believed to be more than seven.

Carrier Oil: (also known as a *base oil*): oil usually from vegetable sources used to dilute essential oils for dermal applications. e.g.: grapeseed, jojoba, safflower, light olive, liquefied coconut, almond, and sunflower

Cold Extraction: the extraction of essential oil from a plant substance without methods that involve heat

Dermal: pertaining to the skin or application/absorption into the body via pores of the skin

Diuretic: increases excretion of urine by stimulating the kidneys

Endocrine: pertaining to the glands and the body's hormonal production. e.g. pancreas, thyroid, adrenals

Endorphin: secretions within the body that can relieve pain and elevate mood. e.g. serotonin, dopamine

Enfleurage: method of obtaining essential oils by soaking plant material in fats. *Does not produce the same concentration as the distillation process.*

Fixative: an essential oil used in perfumery that stabilizes other scent ingredients and makes the fragrance last longer. e.g. frankincense, sandalwood, vetiver

Frequency: a measurable rate of electrical energy constant between two points. Everyone and everything possesses frequency.

Gas Chromatography: a test that breaks down the main chemical components of an essential oil for analysis. Also Enantio-selective gas chromatography (ESGC)

Hydrosol: water penetrated with the scent of a steam-distilled plant substance. e.g. rose or orange flower water

Infusion: herbs, flowers, and other plant substances steeped in water or oil

Integumentary: dermal, pertaining to the skin

Nervine: soothes, balances, and tones the nervous system

Neurotoxin: a substance that can destroy nerve tissue

Neurotransmitters: chemical messengers within the body that regulate mood, pain perception, and vital functions of the body. e.g. acetylcholine, serotonin

pH: acid/alkaline ratio

Resin: a semi-dense liquid exuded from certain trees when the bark is cut or injured, usually concentrated with extraordinary healing properties and aromatic qualities. Some plants also produce resinous material. e.g. frankincense, myrrh

Solvent: a substance capable of dissolving other substances

Synergy: the effect of many components working together as a whole rather than singularly; for the serious essential oil practitioner, synergy is a critical goal in application that can produce the most significant healing effects

Synergistic: works well with

Transdermal: the ability to pass through skin layers

Volatile: Tending to evaporate in a short period of time

<u>Universal Oil:</u> an essential oil that possesses antimicrobial/antibacterial/antiviral/antifungal-like properties. e.g. lavender, clove

Dilution, Blending, and Ratio:

An Easy How-To Guide

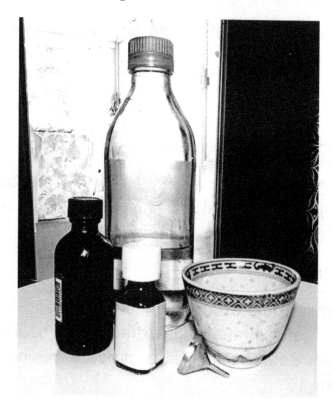

Note: If any essential or carrier oil causes rash or sensitivity, discontinue use and seek a substitution that is well-tolerated.

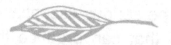

<u>Carrier/Base Oils for Diluting Essential Oils</u>

Recommended Carrier Oils

Apricot Kernel Oil: For all skin types, especially nourishing for sensitive, dry, or mature skin

Coconut Oil: excellent and nutritious oil suitable for all skin types. Coconut oil is solidified at room temperature but is easily liquefied for applications to the skin and for essential oil application. For best quality and integrity of the product, look for virgin or extra virgin coconut oil when purchasing.

Grape Seed (cold pressed): The lightest of all carrier oils, grape seed also has a mild, barely-detectable scent, is rich in antioxidants, and is good for all skin types. Due to its ability to disappear into the skin without a greasy residue, grape seed oil is wonderful oil for dermal blends and massage therapy. However, its shelf life is not as long as jojoba or olive. Store away from sunlight, heat (including heating pads, heat vents, etc.) Recommended for all dermal use including full body massage.

Jojoba Wonderful oil but bear in mind that a little goes a long way. Add approximately 10% to another carrier oil for a lighter base oil. Very soothing to the skin. Recommended for use as a facial oil.

Olive (cold pressed: Although it takes longer for penetration into the skin, light olive oil recommended for baking can be a nice carrier oil. Extra virgin olive oil can be used as a base for small-batch essential oil blends.

Sesame: Very nourishing for the skin, but bear in mind that it is difficult to wash out of sheets and clothing. Residue can turn rancid when in the dryer. Rancidity happens quickly when the bottle is exposed to sunlight or an indoor heat source. Shorter shelf life than other carrier oils. Recommended for facial blends. For massage and use of larger

amounts, use 10% sesame oil combined with a lighter carrier oil such as grapeseed, safflower, or light olive.

Sweet Almond Oil: Excellent oil for all skin types and reduces inflammation.

*Other suitable carrier oils: cold-pressed safflower, cold-pressed sunflower, non-GMO soy, non-GMO corn

RECOMMENDED AMOUNT FOR WHAT

<u>Application to a specific area</u>: **e.g.** sore muscles or application along the spine=1 teaspoon carrier oil

<u>Application for larger area of the body</u>: **e.g.** shoulders or legs=2 teaspoons carrier oil

<u>Full body massage</u>=3 tablespoons carrier oil

RATIO

For diluted blends:

Adults: 2-5 drops of essential oil (s) per teaspoon of carrier oil or unscented lotion / 6-9 drops of essential oil (s) per tablespoon of carrier oil or unscented lotion.

Children: _For Children 0-4 years of age_: Use 1/10 of the recommended amount of essential oils. For example, if you are using an adult ratio of 5 drops essential oil to 1 teaspoon carrier oil, a children's application would be 1 drop essential oil to 1 teaspoon carrier oil. _For ages 5-8 years of age_: 1-3 drops essential oils per teaspoon carrier oil. _For ages 8-12_: 2-4 drops _essential oil per teaspoon carrier oil. For teens up to age 15_: generally half of any adult dose.

Diluting in Aloe Vera Gel: 1-2 drops essential oil per teaspoon of aloe vera gel or juice / 3-4 essential oil per tablespoon of aloe vera gel or juice.

Apply to the body as any other carrier but not recommended for massage. **Tip:** a small amount of supplemental aloe vera gel or juice (obtained as an ingestible supplement in health food stores) can be a conducive carrier for diluting 1 drop of clove essential oil to apply to gums for toothache.

For full body massage:

2-10 drops per tablespoon of carrier oil, unscented lotion, or massage cream, depending upon preferences and which essential oils are used. Stronger essential oils can be used the most sparingly because a little goes a long way. For children's massage, use the minimum recommended amount (1-2 drops for young children, 3-4 for older children.)

For neat (undiluted) application:

Adults: For undiluted application to the soles of the feet, use 3-4 drops of essential oil maximum *per foot.* If you use more than one essential oil, layer the oils and divide the number accordingly without exceeding 8 drops total.

Children: Use 1 drop essential oil *per sole* of the foot.

Tip: The easiest way to apply essential oils neat to the soles of the feet is to simply place an index finger over an essential oil bottle, invert the bottle, and then turn right-side up. The amount of essential oil dispensed on your finger should equal 1 drop. Be sure to allow oils to be absorbed before putting on shoes and socks.

DILUTING BLENDS WITH CARRIER OIL

What You Will Need

Carrier oil

Essential oils of choice

Small ceramic or glass cup OR an empty 1 ounce glass bottle

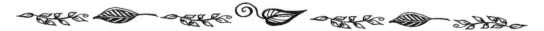

Measuring spoon

Small funnel (optional)

What to do

Basic Template:

1. <u>For Immediate use</u>: Pour carrier oil into a small cup by spoonful.

   <u>To store for multiple uses</u>: To make half-an-ounce or a one ounce bottle blend, measure the amount by tablespoon using a small funnel pre-measure using a salad oil pourer/dispenser. **Tip:** To maintain the integrity of your essential oils and blends, only use colored bottles (amber or cobalt blue) which prevent natural and artificial lights from dissipating potency. Keep empty essential oil bottles to use again for your own blends. See Resources for suppliers of bottles, funnels, pipettes, etc.

2. Add essential oils to a cup or to a bottle drop by drop. Use the minimal amount of essential oil in cases of sensitive skin. **Tip:** Essential oils come out of the bottle with varying speed- lavender, geranium, chamomile, and citrus oils tend to come out very quickly while oils such as myrrh and patchouli are slower. Sometimes bottle droppers vary as well, and the inverted type can be temperamental. No worries if a few drops more than intended come out of the bottle; simply add a trifling bit more of carrier oil in cases of sensitive skin or use on children. On the other hand, if you can't get an essential oil to emerge from the bottle, shake it out with a little force.

3. If blending for one-time use in a cup, swirl ingredients in your cup with gentle, circular hand motions. If using a bottle, cap tightly and hold the bottle between the palms of your hands and gently roll it back and forth. Some aromatherapists prefer mixing oils this way and do not

turn the bottle upside down and right-side up while others use both methods. I personally use both, swirling between the palms of my hands before turning the bottle upside down and right-side up one or two times at the end. **Tip:** Keep in a cool place and out of direct sunlight.

Diluted Cream Blends for Bodywork:

Combine 4-6 drops* of essential oil per tablespoon of unscented lotion or cream; stir together in a small cup with index finger. *For Children: Always use half of the recommended amount per tablespoon. **Tip:** To add essential oils to a bottle of lotion for multiple uses in the treatment room, add approximately 10-15 drops essential oil to the bottle of lotion and mix well in circular motions with a chop stick. Recommended essential oils: lavender, Roman chamomile, or peppermint.

Synergy: *The Heart of Aromatic Medicine*

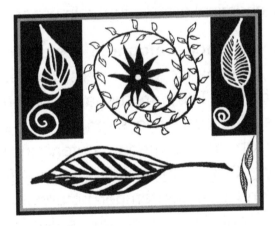

The goal of the everyday user of essential oils is often the same as the professional aromatherapist or massage therapist: becoming proficient in choosing which oils to blend together for a desired effect. It is a beautiful and studious journey that only becomes more valuable and effective over the years but one that does not need to be daunting.

Synergistic blending of essential oils begins with an aromatic palette, much

like a painter works with color and a musician with notes on the scale. Knowing how to choose oils for blends begins with *knowing the properties* of the essential oils, *accessing individual needs* at the moment, and melding *factual* and *intuitive* ability. Each essential oil possesses a frequency, and when combined effectively with others for a specific purpose, resonates with harmonic energies. This harmony enters our bodies and raises our own frequency; every malady, be it physical or emotional, also holds a frequency, and when a certain malady comes in contact with the higher frequency of essential oil synergy, our bodies shift toward balance.

Everyone is different and every physical body individual, therefore results might vary from person to person, and some oils and blends work for some better than others. Essential oils have many properties; there are many to choose from, so it is recommended to try more than one formula and more than one essential oil to find the right match for you at a particular time.

Chemical Components: A Brief Overview

The *major* chemical groups found in essential oils are:

Monoterpenes / monoterpene alcohols restore equilibrium within the body, create vibratory resonance within cells, and are believed to be the most therapeutic in action. They are usually non-irritating, have uplifting and pleasing aromas, and can have strong immune-boosting properties. Essential oils with high monoterpene content include grapefruit 94%, tangerine 94%, orange 90%, lemon 89%, balsam fir 84%, and angelica 76%. Monoterpenes and alcohols temper potentially irritating compounds within an essential oil and work with others like a support system that brings harmony to the body.

Sesquiterpenes reprogram destructive cellular patterns, bring oxygen to the tissues including the brain, and possess deeply relaxing properties which can nourish the nervous system. Essential oils with high sesquiterpene content include Atlas cedarwood 98%, vetiver 97%, spikenard 93%, sandalwood 90%, and black pepper 74%.

Phenols are powerful compounds that initiate healing and combat bacterial, viral, and fungal invaders; they also fight parasites, heavy metals, toxic accumulation of pharmaceutical drugs, and petrochemicals. They are aggressive in the healing process in order for monoterpenes and sesquiterpenes to kick in and do their job. Oils high in phenolic content should be used sparingly due to their potency. Essential oils high in phenols include <u>anise</u> 93%, <u>birch</u> 90%, <u>basil</u> 83%, <u>clove</u> 80%, and <u>oregano</u> 70%.

In an ideal synergistic essential oil blend, there is a balance of these compounds, namely, a harmonic combination of essential oils that possess dominant qualities of each chemical group. I often hear even professional aromatherapists confess that they find it challenging to create a synergistic blend, but I believe this arises from the fact that essential oils share many properties with other essential oils and it can be difficult to choose which ones work best in a particular blend. The final decision should be based upon a person's individual needs at the time, contraindications and sensitivities, and preferences. One does not need to be an advanced medical aromatherapist or an expert in essential oil chemistry to create highly effective and balanced blends, only deep understanding of essential oil properties and hands-on experience using the oils themselves. Over-thinking the synergistic process leaves little room for much-needed intuition, a valuable component in aromatherapy applications, especially when blending for others. After everything is said and done, essential oils possess subtle intelligence and know how to work in our bodies.

Guidelines for Making Synergistic Blends

Synergistic blends can be as simple as two diluted or undiluted essential oils used together or complex as eight essential oils *or more*. Less does not mean more, and the average synergistic blend can have 4-6 essential oils in it.

1. Choose something to be addressed e.g. physical problem or emotional issue.

2. Choose your carrier oil.

3. Decide which essential oils to use depending upon needs and intention; evaluate physical symptoms and emotional symptoms (if applicable.) You may wish to not only address the symptoms at hand but also the possible factors contributing to or causing the symptoms. For example, if you are experiencing stomach or intestinal discomfort during hormonal shifts, creating a blend for hormonal balance might resolve the belly distress. To be sure, use essential oils for the symptoms as well as "the bigger picture."

4. Essential oils have multiple uses and share many properties with each other; learn to not only trust your acquired knowledge but to trust your intuition when undecided about which essential oils to use; also make decisions on aroma preferences when it comes down to two or more oils that may be appropriate for what is being addressed.

5. Do not forget contraindications and find substitutes when applicable.

6. Add essential oils one at a time, counting drops and writing down your formula. Keeping notes ensures accuracy in case you want to use that blend again.

7. If making a blend to use immediately, apply it as soon as possible and do not leave it out to be exposed to the air longer than twenty minutes, especially when using resinous essential oils such as frankincense and myrrh or citrus oils such as lemon. If storing in a bottle, be sure to cap tightly and swirl bottle between the palms of the hands to mix well.

Tip: If using synergy for neat application to the soles of the feet, apply one essential oil at a time, layering the oils.

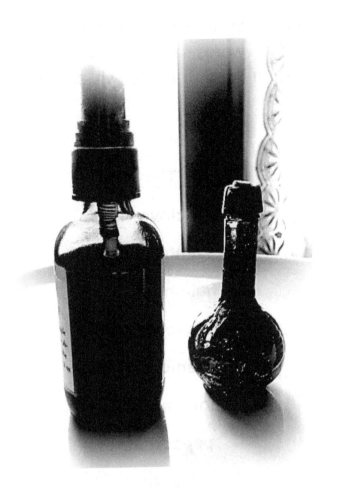

Which Oils for What:

A Preliminary Go-To Guide

UNIVERSAL OILS

Definition:

essential oils that possess antiseptic, antibacterial, antiviral, and antifungal-like properties. In other words, essential oils that do it all and are recommended to have on hand at home, while traveling, and in the First-Aid kit.

What They Are

clove

eucalyptus radiata

helichrysum

lavender

organic lemon

lemon eucalyptus

peppermint

tea tree

white thyme

Primary Uses

-strengthening the immune system to prevent illness (*all of the above*)

-colds, flu, and infections (*all of the above*)

-First-Aid (*lavender, tea tree, helichrysum*)

HOW TO USE UNIVERSAL OILS

For better immunity: All Universal Oils (*clove, eucalyptus radiata, lavender, organic lemon, lemon eucalyptus, tea tree, white thyme*)

Applied undiluted to the soles of the feet (see page 24), universal oils can be used *singularly or combined* with each other to boost the immune system and prevent illness. They can also be used to minimize the severity or duration of colds, flu, and other viral infections. If used to boost immunity, do not use a single oil for more than a week, for the body becomes immune and does not respond as well. At week's end, simply switch to another single oil for the full immune-boosting benefits. **e.g.** if you use organic lemon oil for better immunity, after a week, switch to another universal oil such as lavender or clove. Also, pair them together for even better results for strong immune system response during cold/flu season or whenever the body is fighting a bacterial or viral condition.

Suggestions for combinations: lavender & organic lemon / white thyme & lavender / organic lemon & clove / tea tree & organic lemon (See page 196 for more immune-boosting formulas)

Important Tip: Begin using universal oils *a few weeks before* cold and flu season and *continue* to use them throughout the winter and spring to prevent or decrease your chances of getting sick. Prevention is the best approach. Once you are sick, universal oils can help your immune system fight viruses, but not all of them will clear up lung congestion, coughs, or bronchitis. *Exception:* lemon eucalyptus & eucalyptus radiata. See **Primary Oils for Respiratory Health**.

For First-Aid: *lavender, tea tree, helichrysum*

A drop or two of lavender essential oil can be applied to a cut, scrape, burn, insect sting, or soft tissue injury (strain or sprain), to stop bleeding (cuts), speed healing, and disinfect the area. Lavender is a must-have oil in the First-Aid Kit and on hand for traveling. Think of it as a one-in-all crisis oil.

Lavender, when applied immediately after an injury or fall, will prevent bruising and swelling, lessen pain, and speed up recovery. Lavender and tea tree essential oils, singularly or combined, will also kill nail and skin fungus. A drop or two of tea tree can be applied daily to a cut after the healing process has begun.

Helichrysum is also an excellent essential oil to apply to any injury from cuts to burns, sprained ankles to strained muscles. It can be applied neat (undiluted) to the area. For older injuries, dilution is recommended.

First-Aid Spray

Add *7 drops lavender & 3 drops tea tree essential oil* to a small spray bottle ¾ filled with distilled water. Spray onto cuts, scrapes, wounds, and burns before applying bandage. Use First-Aid spray 1-2x daily.

For Toothache: 1 drop clove essential oil added to ½ a teaspoon of aloe vera gel and mixed well can be applied to the gum for toothache or before and after dental treatment. Clove is analgesic and will reduce pain considerably.

Seasonal Allergies/Food Sensitivities:

1 undiluted drop of lavender and organic lemon essential oil to the palms of the hands and rubbed together can have an antihistamine effect, especially for food sensitivities such as dairy as well as seasonal allergies in some individuals. **Recommendation**: apply every half hour for 2 hours.

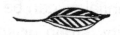

PRIMARY OILS FOR RESPIRATORY HEALTH**

eucalyptus (*do not use if asthmatic*)

lemon eucalyptus (*do not use if asthmatic*)

peppermint (*do not use if asthmatic*)

organic lemon

frankincense

pine needle

Primary Uses

-Coughs, congestion, sinus, and lung infections

For Respiratory and Sinus Conditions Including Pneumonia:

Diffuse any of these oils or any combination of these oils into the air and/or dilute and rub onto the chest (all except lemon essential oil) to break up congestion and dry up watery coughs. Use as a steam inhalation application to open the sinuses or address acute or chronic sinus infections (See page 243 for inhalation recipes.) These primary respiratory allies open the bronchial pathways for easier breathing and increase oxygen in the blood. Organic lemon applied to the soles of the feet or diffused into the air via nebulizer is a powerful ally against pneumonia. Eucalyptus, peppermint, frankincense, balsam fir, and pine needle essential oils are also effective and pleasant when added to a healing bath.

Caution: Do not use lemon essential oil in the bath, for it can irritate the skin. *If asthmatic, avoid all eucalyptus, mint, and camphor oils and use frankincense, balsam fir, or pine needle instead unless it is certain that menthol can be tolerated without problems.*

Recommended Combinations for Chest Rubs: frankincense & balsam fir / eucalyptus & pine needle / lemon eucalyptus & peppermint

Recommended Combinations for Diffusion via Nebulizer: organic lemon & lemon eucalyptus / peppermint & eucalyptus

Recommended Combinations for the Bath: pine needle & eucalyptus / peppermint & balsam fir / frankincense & balsam fir

PRIMARY OILS FOR ANXIETY & STRESS

basil

frankincense

lavender

neroli

ylang ylang

Primary Uses

-balancing the nervous system

-anxiety and panic attacks

-everyday stress

For Everyday Stress: Use any inhalation method, single oils or in combination with each other. Also apply neat to the soles of the feet (see page 24 for details.) Good combinations for dermal use are: lavender &

ylang ylang / lavender & frankincense / neroli & ylang ylang used on the soles of the feet or diluted as a massage oil. Can also be used in the bath (see page 248 for details.)

For Anxiety and Panic Attacks: Use any inhalation method (see page 221 for details), especially lavender and frankincense essential oils on a tissue for quick results. Ylang ylang and neroli combined and inhaled make a powerful, non-drowsy combination with wonderful sedative properties that will stop trembling, shaking, and adrenaline rushes almost immediately. Mixing oils into bath salts for a foot bath is an effective way to relieve anxiety and stress. *When panic and anxiety attacks are stubborn and all else fails, try a drop of basil on the palm of the hand and inhale.* Diluted dermal applications of essential oils will help prevent or lessen the frequency of attacks. For this purpose, combine and dilute: lavender, frankincense/ ylang ylang or neroli, lavender, & frankincense

Important Tip: Apply along the spine every morning and evening.

For Better Sleep: Use any inhalation method (see page 200 for details), especially lavender, neroli, and ylang ylang singularly or combined. Oils can also be spritzed onto a pillow case or sheets.

For Calming a Nervous Belly: Inhale lavender and frankincense for approximately 10 minutes. Also dilute and apply along the spine. Basil is also a good choice for some people and can be inhaled for a minute or two.

For job Interviews, Exams, and Public Speaking: Inhale basil to balance the nervous system, quell jitters, sharpen memory, and boost confidence.

For Arguments, Intense Emotions, and Adrenaline Rushes: A drop of ylang ylang on a tissue or the palm of the hand will help the nervous system reset after emotional turmoil or angry outbursts. Combine ylang ylang with neroli for even better results; both oils can be diluted or combined and applied to the skin along the spine, the arms, and the chest to regulate adrenaline. This combination is also wonderful for women during hormonal shifts when heart palpitations and adrenaline rushes are

common. In this case, inhalation works immediately while dermal applications may prevent or lessen frequency of occurrences.

PRIMARY OILS FOR DECREASING PAIN

balsam fir

eucalyptus

ginger

helichrysum

lavender

peppermint

pine needle

spearmint

Primary Uses

-relieving soft-tissue pain related to over-exertion

-muscle strains, sprains, and bruises

-lessening osteoarthritis and rheumatoid arthritis pain; managing painful flares associated with chronic pain disorders including fibromyalgia and myofascial pain syndrome

-pain associated with influenza

-preventing muscle soreness after workouts or physical exertion

-to lessen or prevent bruising after falls and injuries

For Over-Exertion, Muscle Strains, and Sprains: Any of the above-mentioned oils singularly or used in combination with each other (2-4 oils may be combined for maximum benefit) diluted in carrier oil can be applied immediately after a workout or injury to lessen pain, bring circulation to the soft tissues and nutrition to the cells. Applying lavender after a fall or impact-injury will lessen or prevent bruising and swelling if applied undiluted and copiously to the area. Apply 2x a day for up to three days after injury to prevent swelling and bruising. Pine needle or balsam fir essential oil combined with peppermint oil and diluted makes an excellent go-to blend for muscle soreness of any kind. Knee injuries and chronic knee pain respond very well to applications of eucalyptus oil used singularly or combined with peppermint.

Important Tip: Contrary to recommended application, essential oils can be applied directly to the knee without dilution unless irritation (itchiness or other unpleasant skin reactions) develops. In that case, dilute the essential oils.

For Osteoarthritis Pain: Balsam fir combined with eucalyptus and diluted makes an effective blend for the pain of osteoarthritis.

For Rheumatoid Arthritis Pain: Balsam fir or helichrysum diluted and used singularly or combined makes an effective blend for the pain of rheumatoid arthritis.

For Fibromyalgia or Pain Syndromes: Ginger essential oil is very warming, antiflammatory-like in action, and brings deep relief in cases of pain syndromes such as fibromyalgia. It can also be combined with balsam fir, pine needle, or spearmint. These oils can be helpful when added to the bath via bath salts. **Recommendation:** Apply any of the above combinations diluted 1-2x a day

See page 205 for detailed recipes for pain management

anise (*Pimpinella anisum*)

sweet basil

bergamot

cacao

grapefruit

lemon

lemongrass

peppermint

rose absolute, rose otto

sweet orange

Primary Uses

-for mild-moderate symptoms of depression

-for Monday morning blues

-for premenstrual and other hormonally-related 'blues'

-to lessen some symptoms of mild-moderate S.A.D. (Seasonal Affective Disorder)

-to lift the spirits and improve mood

For Starting the Day on a Positive Note: 1 or 2 drops of essential oil on a tissue or inhaled as a steam can help stimulate feel-good endorphins. These recommended oils can be used singularly or combined. Good

essential oil combinations for beginning the day in a better frame of mind and more energy include: grapefruit & tangerine / bergamot & lemongrass / peppermint & basil / cacao & sweet orange / lemon & star anise*. Rose essential oil used singularly helps the brain produce more dopamine, the neurotransmitter and hormone responsible for good mood, fortitude, and a hopeful attitude.

Tip: A few drops sprinkled on a wash cloth or sponge can be placed in the shower; the aroma fills the tub/shower as the water heats up, and a fragrant steam can be inhaled. See detailed recipes for mood and emotions on page 221.

Caution: Individuals with epilepsy or who are prone to seizures should not inhale star anise or anise seed essential oil.

PRIMARY OILS FOR DIGESTIVE TROUBLES

anise (*Pimpinella anisum*)

cardamom

ginger

peppermint

spearmint

<u>Primary Uses:</u>

-ease intestinal distress (pain, rumbling)

-lessen gas and bloating

- nausea

-lessen or resolve acute diarrhea

- symptoms of indigestion

-stimulate sluggish appetite

-lessen constipation and stimulate peristalsis of the muscles of the digestive tract

-decrease or resolve candida overgrowth in the intestines

-to boost good flora in the intestines after antibiotic use

For Indigestion, Bloating, Pain, Flatulence, and Other Digestive Upsets: Peppermint essential oil is the go-to oil for any stomach and intestinal issue. Add up to 3-5 drops of the essential oil in 1-2 teaspoons carrier oil or unscented lotion and apply to abdomen 1-2x a day. If skin is sensitive, use 2-3 drops of essential oil diluted in carrier oil or lotion.

For Diarrhea from Diet, Stress, or Hormonal Upset: Add 5 drops peppermint and 2 drops lavender essential oils diluted in 1 teaspoon of carrier oil or unscented lotion and apply to the navel/lower abdomen 1-3x a day 4 hours apart.

For Diarrhea from Bacterial or Viral Infection: Add 2 drops peppermint, 2 drops patchouli, 2 drops sweet orange, and 1 drop clove essential oil diluted in 1 teaspoon of carrier oil or unscented lotion and apply to the navel/lower abdomen 1-3x a day 4 hours apart.

For Occasional Constipation: Add 1-2 drops of ginger essential oil to 1 teaspoon of carrier oil or unscented lotion and apply to abdomen 1-2x a day.

For Nausea and/or Vomiting: A speck of spearmint or peppermint essential oil under the tongue will decrease nausea within minutes or even seconds. Touching the point of a wooden toothpick on the bottle of

essential oil equals the appropriate amount.   Use when needed up to 4x within an hour.

For Acid Indigestion, Discomfort after Eating, Belching, or Hiccups: A speck of spearmint, peppermint, or anise seed essential oil applied under the tongue will help ease discomfort after eating. Touching the point of a wooden toothpick on the bottle of essential oil equals the appropriate amount. **Tip:** Using this method with spearmint essential oil is wonderfully effective for heartburn and hiccups.

To Boost Good Flora in the Intestines After Taking Antibiotics or for Systemic Candida/Yeast: Apply 2 drops lavender, 1 drop tea tree, and 2 drops clove essential oil undiluted to the soles of the feet every evening before bed. Do this for two weeks. For chronic systemic yeast issues, use this method for two weeks and then stop for a week; repeat as needed. Drink plenty of water throughout the day to flush toxins from the system.

Primary Oils for Skin Health

carrot seed

frankincense

helichrysum

lavender

Roman chamomile

rose hip

rosewood

tea tree

Primary Uses

-First-Aid

-to clear pimples and decrease irritation

-to moisturize the skin

-to decrease excessive oil

-to nourish mature skin

-to decrease scars

-promote healing

-to decrease inflammation

-to treat insect bites

-decrease age spots

-possible skin cancer prevention

-for shingles

-for fungal/yeast rash

For Healing of Cuts, Scrapes, and Burns: Undiluted lavender essential oil applied to cuts, scrapes, and burns can speed healing and bring nutrition to the skin. It will also disinfect the area. Apply 1 drop up to 3x daily for up to five days if needed.

To Minimize Scars and Keloid Scars: Add 2 drops frankincense and 2 drops carrot seed essential oil to ½-1 teaspoon of carrier oil and apply to the scar daily.

As a Moisturizer: Add 5 drops carrot seed, 4 drops rose hip, and 1 drop of lavender essential oil to 1 ounce of liquefied coconut or olive oil and apply to skin daily. For mature skin, add 1-2 drops frankincense essential oil.

To Decrease Age Spots: Add 1 drop carrot seed and 2 drops frankincense essential oil to a teaspoon of carrier oil and apply to the skin. Do this two times daily until desired results.

For Oily Skin: Fill a small spritzer/spray bottle with distilled water and add 4 drops of ylang ylang, 1 drop lavender, and 1 drop geranium essential oil. Shake well before each use, close eyes, and spritz on the face after washing. Can be applied before bed and in the morning before applying make-up.

For Dry Skin: *Hydrating water method*: Fill a small spritzer/spray bottle with distilled water and add 4 drops of lavender, 3 drops frankincense, and 1 drop geranium essential oil. Shake well before each use, close eyes, and spritz on the face after washing. Can be applied before bed and in the morning before applying make-up. *Oil-Based Moisturizer*: Add 1 drop lavender, 1 drop frankincense, and 1 drop geranium essential oils to approximately 1 teaspoon of liquefied coconut, olive, or sesame oil and apply morning and evening. This can be used under make-up after the skin absorbs it. *Aloe-Based Moisturizer*: Add 1 drop lavender and 1 drop frankincense essential oil to 1 teaspoon of aloe vera juice or gel and apply morning and evening. This can be used under make-up after the skin absorbs it.

For Red and Irritated Skin: Add 1 drop lavender and 1 drop Roman chamomile essential oil to aloe juice or gel, mix well, and apply to skin up to 2x a day.

For Skin Cancers and/or Prevention of: Add 3 drops frankincense and 3 drops lavender essential oil to 1 teaspoon extra virgin olive oil and apply to pre-cancerous or cancerous skin growths or lesions up to 3x a day. Alternate combination: Add 3 drops frankincense and 2 drops lavender, and 1 drop rosewood essential oils to 1 teaspoon extra virgin olive oil and apply to pre-cancerous or cancerous skin growths or lesions up to 3x a day. **Caution:** *This application is not to be substituted for conventional medical treatment. Use essential oil application in conjunction with traditional medical treatment for best results.*

For Pimples: Apply a bit of tea tree essential oil to blemishes 2x a day-after washing in the morning and the evening. You can also add 2 drops lavender and 3 drops tea tree essential oil to a small spritzer/spray bottle of distilled water. Shake well before use and spritz onto pimples 2x daily after washing in the morning and in the evening.

For Insect Bites: Apply a drop of lavender and/or tea tree essential oil straight from the bottle onto insect bites to decrease irritation, inflammation, discomfort, and itching. Up to 4x a day.

For Shingles Rash: Add 2 drops ravensara, 1 drop frankincense, 1 drop rosewood, 1 drop lavender, and 1 drop geranium essential oil in 1 tablespoon of nourishing carrier oil such as grapeseed oil or light olive oil. Apply to shingles rash 2x a day, morning and evening. **Tip:** Best used in conjunction with application of essential oils to the soles of the feet to address systemically: apply 1 drop clove, 1 drop tea tree, and 3 drops lemon eucalyptus essential oils to each sole of the foot 2x a day for a week.

For Fungal/Yeast Rash: 2-3 drops rosewood and 1 drop lavender essential oil to a teaspoon of carrier oil and apply to rash 2x a day. For nail fungus, apply 1 drop tea tree and 1 drop lavender essential oil undiluted (neat) to nail bed 2x a day. For athlete's foot, add 3 drops tea tree, 3 drops lavender, and 3 drops rosewood essential oil to warm water and soak feet once a day. Do not rinse and dry feet well.

Tip: If rosewood essential oil is difficult to find or if you choose to not use this oil obtained from endangered trees, you can substitute with geranium essential oil.

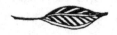

Primary oils for Better Sleep

Atlas cedarwood

lavender

neroli

rosewood

spikenard

ylang ylang

Primary Uses

-to calm the body and relax tense muscles

-naturally increase melatonin

For Better Sleep: Put 2 drops ylang ylang and 1 drop lavender essential oil to a tissue, fold, and inhale for 10-15 minutes before going to sleep. Best used in conjunction with dermal application: apply 2 drops Atlas cedarwood, 1 drop spikenard, and 2 drops lavender to the soles of the feet right before sleep. Alternate dermal combinations: 3 drops lavender and 3 drops rosewood essential oil for soles of the feet OR 3 drops lavender and 2 drops Roman chamomile to soles of the feet right before sleep.

Essential Oils Considered Safe for Children and Babies

bergamot (Citrus bergamia)

cedarwood, Atlas (Cedrus atlantica)

chamomile, Roman (Chamaemelum nobile)

frankincense (Boswellia carteri)

geranium (Pelargonium graveolens)

lavender (Lavandula angustifolia)

mandarin (Citrus reticulata)

marjoram (Origanum majorana)

orange (Citrus aurantium)

rosalina (Melaleuca ericifolia)

rose otto (Rosa damascena)

rosewood (Aniba rosaeodora)

sandalwood (Santalum album)

tea tree (Melaleuca alternifolia)

ylang ylang (Cananga odorata)

II

THE ESSENTIAL OIL PROFILES

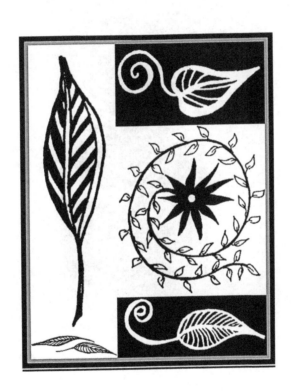

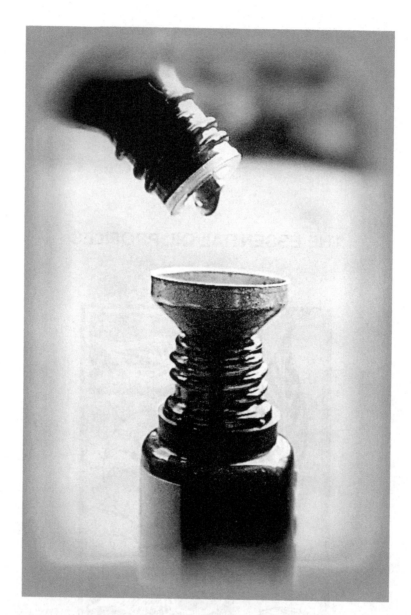

Essential Oil Reference Guide

Allspice (Pimenta officinalus)

Scent: spicy, warm

Clinical Uses: sinusitis/ viral and bacterial infection / flatulence and indigestion / muscle spasms / pain / depression / nervous exhaustion

Body Systems Affected: immune, gastrointestinal, musculoskeletal, respiratory, endocrine, nervous

Inhalation Effect: uplifting for mood and outlook

Dermal Effect: for soft tissue pain (muscles, joints, ligaments) / strengthened immune response / general fatigue / good for coughs when diluted and applied to throat and chest

Practical Uses: antiseptic for household cleaning

Vibrational Influence: encourages receptivity to positive change, abundance, and self-expression

Emotional Influence: promotes self-esteem / inspires courage to try after failure / revives hope / gives a sense of security / helps release unexpressed grief and shame

Synergistic to: clove, ginger, bay (Pimenta racemosa)

Chakra Correspondence: root, sacral/navel, solar plexus heart

Cosmetic Use: used in perfumery

Source and Parts Used: berries from the tree

Amber (see Storax)

Amyris (Amyris balsamifera)

Scent: soft musk with sweet, earthy undertones

Clinical Uses: nervousness due to stress and deadlines/ emotional exhaustion

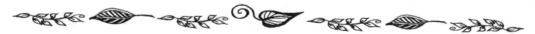

Body Systems Affected: nervous system / limbic brain

Inhalation Effect: calms scattered thoughts and frazzled nerves / enhances creativity

Dermal Effect: calms physical symptoms of anxiety

Practical Uses: lovely to put a few drops on pillow case or tissue

Vibrational Influence: clears toxic psychic debris in the energy field / resonates with the Sacred Feminine

Emotional Influence: instills trust in the flow of life

Synergistic to: sandalwood, vetiver

Chakra Correspondence: heart, root

Cosmetic Use: a fixative in perfumery and for musky undertones / added to skin care designed for mature skin

Source and Parts Used: wood from the tree

Tip: Amrys essential oil can be substituted for expensive and endangered sandalwood

Angelica Root (Angelica archangelica)

Scent: root-like and sweet

Clinical Uses: menstrual disorders/ nervous conditions and nervous exhaustion / respiratory weakness and infection / gastritis and stomach problems from nervous origin / strengthening of the body after illness, childbirth, or grief / anorexia nervosa

Body Systems Affected: endocrine, nervous, immune

Inhalation Effect: calms an over-stimulated sympathetic nervous system / soothes inflamed sinuses / lifts the mood

Dermal Effect: helps to balance women's hormones especially during PMS and after childbirth / strengthens and tones female reproductive system / eases respiratory ailments / supports the adrenals

Practical Uses: N/A

Vibrational Influence: strengthens the energy field and is especially useful for empaths and anyone who works in medical, holistic, or caregiving fields / encourages resolution regarding acknowledged or forgotten traumatic memories / connects one's spirit to the finer spiritual realms / resonates with the angelic kingdoms

Emotional Influence: instills calm and sense of well-being / inspires hope / lifts the spirit from depression and feelings of defeat / useful during times of grief, loss, and hopelessness

Synergistic to: geranium, rosewood, spruce, vetiver

Chakra Correspondence: root, sacral/navel, solar plexus, heart

Cosmetic Use: N/A except for a deep, earthy base note/fixative in perfumery

Source and Parts Used: root of the plant

Caution: *Do not use while pregnant; some sources recommend that individuals with diabetes avoid angelica essential oil. Avoid direct sunlight or tanning beds for 24 hours after dermal application.*

Tip: This rather expensive oil can be purchased in affordable diluted form and possesses the same properties and pleasant scent.

Anise a.k.a. Aniseed (Pimpinella anisum)

Scent: licorice-like and confectionary, similar to fennel and star anise

Clinical Uses: hormonal stimulation in women, especially prolactin and estrogen / intestinal discomfort, sluggish digestion, colic / congestion / menstrual pain / sexual impotence / headache / painful menstruation / women's hormonal headaches

Body Systems Affected: gastrointestinal, reproductive, nervous/limbic brain, respiratory

Inhalation Effect: elevates mood / lessens nausea

Dermal Effect: increases lactation in nursing mothers / aids digestion, soothes intestinal extremes (diarrhea or constipation) / estrogen-like for menopausal discomforts / can be rubbed on the belly with a carrier oil or lotion for belly ache or intestinal distress

Practical Uses: a tiny drop or a speck on the finger and rubbed under the tongue will freshen breath, allay nausea, and promote digestion / antiseptic for household cleaning

Vibrational Influence: cleanses sadness, despair, and festering anger from the energy field

Emotional Influence: inspires hope / lifts mood, lessens fear / calms nervous-related physical ailments

Synergistic to: sweet fennel seed, star anise, spearmint, peppermint, cardamom, ginger

Chakra Correspondence: sacral/navel, solar plexus

Cosmetic Use: flavoring in toothpastes, mouthwashes, and as a top note in perfumery

Source and Parts Used: seeds from the plant

Caution: *According to some sources, anise essential oil should be not used dermally by people who have or have had estrogen-dependent cancer. Women with endometriosis or a history of endometriosis should not use anise essential oil dermally. Individuals on blood thinners should avoid dermal use of anise essential oil. Anise (Pimpinella anisum) is not the same as Star Anise (Illicium verum). Each essential oil comes from two different sources and despite sharing similarities, offer different benefits and serious contraindications. Some essential oil companies often combine the two essential oils and sell them as Anise. Be discerning and look for the Latin botanical name if you are using anise or star anise for clinical dermal applications. See Caution for Star Anise for contraindications for liver disease, alcoholism, etc.*

Anise, Star (Illicium verum)

Scent: licorice-like, bright and pungent

Clinical Uses: bronchitis / colds and flu / weak appetite / queasy stomach / sluggish digestion

Body Systems Affected: respiratory, gastrointestinal

Inhalation Effect: brightens the mood / calms agitation and worry

Dermal Effect: lessens phlegm and congestion of the lungs and sinuses

Practical Uses: makes a lovely addition to household cleaners and room sprays

Vibrational Influence: brightens the energy field of places and people

Emotional Influence: clears away feelings of defeat / instills a sense of renewal

Synergistic to: sweet fennel, coriander, cardamom

Chakra Correspondence: sacral/navel, heart, brow

Cosmetic Use: added to cosmetics and fragrances for a confectionary top note

Source and Parts Used: seeds from the evergreen tree

Caution: *According to some sources, star anise essential oil should be not used dermally by people who have or have had estrogen-dependent cancer. Individuals on blood thinners or paracetamol should avoid dermal use of star anise essential oil. Avoid star anise essential oil in cases of liver disease, alcoholism, liver disease, and endometriosis. Star anise is considered to have narcotic properties in large doses and can dangerously slow down circulation which can lead to brain damage. Do not use excessively via dermal use or inhalation. Star anise (Illicium verum) is not the same as Anise Pimpinella anisum). Each essential oil comes from two different sources and despite sharing similarities, offer different benefits and serious contraindications. Some essential oil companies combine the two essential oils and sell them as Anise. Be discerning and look for the Latin botanical name if you are using anise or star anise for clinical dermal applications.*

Basil (Ocimum basilicum)

Scent: pungent, sweet, bright and herbaceous

Clinical Uses: balancing the nervous system / fatigue from boredom and drudgery / impaired memory / herpes and shingles / mental overwork / ADD / oxygen deficiency in brain / severe anxiety when nothing else stops a panic attack / apathy, depression, melancholy / migraine headaches / Parkinson's Disease / addiction recovery and cravings associated with addictions

Body Systems Affected: nervous, endocrine, immune

Inhalation Effect: elevates mood / instills ambition and motivation / jumpstarts the body on Monday mornings and during afternoon slumps / improves memory and mental clarity- great before taking a test, studying, or giving a presentation / calms scattered thoughts in cases of ADD & ADHD / increases oxygen to the brain / may halt a panic attack with a few whiffs when all else fails / may be helpful for Parkinson's Disease / helpful in boosting neurotransmitters, therefore capable of reducing cravings associated with addiction including non-substance addictions like gambling, spending, and sex

Dermal Effect: helps immune system fight the herpes virus / tones the nervous system and acts as a stimulant or a restorative depending upon the body's immediate needs / helps to build energy reserves or life force in organ systems / may prevent or minimize migraine headaches / may be helpful for Parkinson's disease

Practical Uses: antiseptic for household cleaning / study aid / air freshener / lessens stings of insect bites when diluted and applied in small amounts

Vibrational Influence: instills hope on a cellular, physical level / supports adrenal life force / encourages receptivity to self-worth, courage, and good outcomes to endeavors / clears the energy field of people and places

Emotional Influence: opens the psyche to experiencing more joy / eases emotional exhaustion and restores hope

Synergistic to: geranium, rosewood, peppermint, juniper berry

Chakra Correspondence: root, solar plexus, throat

Cosmetic Use: minimal amount in perfumery for a 'green' top note

Source and Parts Used: leaves and stems from the aromatic plant

Tip: Inhaling basil can be almost immediate in stopping severe anxiety or panic, especially when the body reacts to triggers with nausea. Good oil to keep on hand at all times, even bedside, for people suffering from panic attacks, for it often works when other remedies fail. *Use sparingly and do not inhale for periods longer than a few minutes, for basil can easily overstimulate the nervous system and counteract its benefits.*

Bay a.k.a. (Pimenta racemosa)

Scent: spicy bay rum

Clinical Uses: sore muscles / muscle strains and sprains / colds and flu / sluggish circulation / anorexia nervosa / tonsillitis

Body Systems Affected: musculoskeletal, immune, nervous/limbic brain

Inhalation Effect: provides a boost of energy when needed / clears the mind for better mental focus

Dermal Effect: stimulates immune system / stimulates circulation / helpful for eating disorders

Practical Uses: nice scent to use for clothes when sprinkled generously onto a damp wash cloth and added with wet clothes in the dryer

Vibrational Influence: helps one to be realistic while pursuing goals

Emotional Influence: fosters confidence and hope for a brighter future

Synergistic to: black pepper, ginger

Chakra Correspondence: root, solar plexus

Cosmetic Use: key ingredient in colognes commonly marketed as "Bay Rum" / added to shampoos to control dandruff

Source and Parts Used: leaves from the West Indian tree, bay rum

Caution: *Do not use bay essential oil if you have or have had prostate cancer, kidney or liver problems, or hemophilia. Do not use bay essential*

oil if you are on anticoagulant medication. Use diluted and sparingly in massage for muscle pain.

Tip: do not confuse Bay essential oil with Bay Laurel; they are from two distinctly different botanical sources. *See Caution for Bay Laurel regarding blood thinners, hemophilia, and narcotic properties.*

<u>Bay Laurel</u> (Laurus nobilis)

a.k.a. Laurel or by its botanical Latin name

Scent: spicy, herbaceous with spicy overtones

Clinical Uses: serious viral infections / lymphatic congestion / swellings / shows significant action against SARS coronavirus / combats Staph, E. coli, and Strep / nerve regeneration / malaria

Body Systems Affected: immune, respiratory, circulatory, endocrine

Inhalation Effect: effective against cold and flu when diffused into the air via nebulizer / decreases pain of sinus headache / *Caution: Use sparingly and not close to mucus membranes—inhale one drop on a folded tissue or use nebulizer to disperse into the air*

Dermal Effect: strong antiviral-like properties / strengthens immunity / effective against malaria / decreases congestion of swollen lymph nodes / recommended for osteoarthritis and rheumatoid arthritis / muscle and joint pain, and nerves in need of regeneration / stimulating to the adrenals / *Caution: use only on the soles of the feet for dermal use*

Practical Uses: insect repellant

Vibrational Influence: clears away confusion and fosters clarity / inspires creativity and self-expression / opens and awakens finer spiritual senses / detaches negative influences from the energy field and psyche

Emotional Influence: increases receptivity to change / stimulates creativity and self-expression

Synergistic to: allspice, clove, juniper berry

Chakra Correspondence: throat, sacral/navel

Cosmetic Use: spicy, "masculine" notes in perfumery and soaps

Source and Parts Used: leaves and twigs of the shrub

Caution: *Use only in moderation. Bay laurel has narcotic properties due to its methyl eugenol content. Do not use if on blood thinners or have hemophilia. Do not use in massage, even small amounts are not recommended.*

Tip: do not confuse *Bay Laurel* essential oil with Bay. They are from two distinctly different botanical sources.

Benzoin (Styrax benzoin)

a.k.a. Onycha and Friar's Balsam

Scent: balsamic with warm vanilla overtones

Clinical Uses: anxiety / lung congestion / depression

Body Systems Affected: nervous, respiratory

Inhalation Effect: breaks up congestion of sinuses and lungs / lifts the tired mind and elevates mood / brings sense of comfort during transition / inspires sensuality

Dermal Effect: calms the nervous system

Practical Uses: antiseptic for household cleaning / scenting the home / nice ingredient for potpourri blends / good oil for meditation

Vibrational Influence: inspires spirituality / protects the energy field / a good oil for anointing during prayer or ritual / stimulates the finer spiritual senses / energetically, provides balm to an individual attempting to heal from past abuse or trauma—especially effective for women / may help an individual overcome fear of loving or being loved

Emotional Influence: grounds the heart in times of passionate intensity / promotes self-love / provides emotional nourishment during times of deep heartache and grief

Synergistic to: sandalwood, amrys, storax, myrrh

Chakra Correspondence: heart, solar-plexus, sacral/navel, root, brow

Cosmetic Use: used as a base note in perfumery / skin balms

Source and Parts Used: resin from the tree

Tip: Benzoin is a key ingredient in high-quality essential oil blends labeled as "amber."

Bergamot (Citrus bergamia)

Scent: sweet and fruity citrus with a bright "green" undertone

Clinical Uses: pancreatic and liver stimulation / sluggish digestion / hypertension / depression / shock / stress-related ailments / nervous heart palpitations / fevers / insomnia

Body Systems Affected: endocrine, gastrointestinal, nervous, circulatory

Inhalation Effect: stimulates dopamine and other endorphins in the brain, thus lifting mental and emotional heaviness / clears the mind for mental work / transforms stagnant energy into free-flowing life force / stimulates appetite / calms nervous system especially stress-related headaches / excellent for weepiness or depression related to female hormonal fluctuations / prevents insomnia if inhaled before sleep

Dermal Effect: stimulates pancreatic secretion and improves liver function / antiseptic for skin issues including acne

Practical Uses: antiseptic for household cleaning / good oil to use before a test, studying, or giving a presentation

Vibrational Influence: increases frequency of the physical body / dissolves fear locked in the energy field, psyche, and bodily tissues

Emotional Influence: revives hope / eases sadness and grief / releases endorphins, calms anxiety especially stage fright / inspires creativity and ambition / helps balance PMS-related mood swings

Synergistic to: geranium, grapefruit, basil

Chakra Correspondence: solar plexus, heart, brow

Cosmetic Use: great for oily and acne-prone skin / helps skin maintain firmness longer / adds a luscious top note to perfumes

Source and Parts Used: cold-pressed fruit peels of the bitter orange also called Seville

Caution: *Individuals on blood thinners should avoid dermal use of bergamot essential oil. Bergamot should not be used prior to direct sun exposure or tanning beds. Severe adverse skin reactions could result. Wait 72 hours to be sure.*

Tip: To avoid photosensitivity, look for *bergaptene-free* essential oil.

Birch, Sweet (Betula lenta)

Scent: similar to root beer and wintergreen, sweet with minty undertones

Clinical Uses: muscular and joint pain / osteoarthritis / adult fever / sinus and lung congestion / sciatica / gout / influenza

Body Systems Affected: musculo-skeletal, respiratory, immune

Inhalation Effect: eases head colds, sinus congestion, and sinus pain / helps break up phlegm in the lungs / *Caution*: intended for short term use only

Dermal Effect*: eases body aches from influenza and colds / helps lessen fibromyalgia pain, osteoarthritis, muscle sprains and sprains / sciatica / diuretic / *Caution*: intended for short term use only and small amounts

Practical Uses: good First-Aid for sprains and strains, short term use only

Vibrational Influence: cleanses the energy field / helps one move into the present time and leave emotional baggage behind / helps restore life force in cases of physical and emotional depletion after periods of prolonged stress

Emotional Influence: clears mental heaviness

Synergistic to: peppermint, eucalyptus

Chakra Correspondence: root

Cosmetic Use: N/A

Source and Parts Used: bark of the tree

Caution: *Individuals on blood thinners should avoid dermal use of birch essential oil. Birch essential oil contains high levels of methyl salicylate, the chemical precursor to aspirin; those allergic to aspirin should not use this essential oil and seek alternatives (e.g. eucalyptus, peppermint, spearmint, ginger, etc.) Birch essential oil should only be used in small amounts on occasion. Avoid regular or long-term use to avoid toxicity.*

Tip: True birch essential oil is rare and often substituted with wintergreen.

Pepper, Black (Piper nigrum)

Scent: spicy, warm peppercorns

Clinical Uses: spleen support / poor circulation / everyday aches and pains / overall sluggishness of the body / fatigue from boredom and monotonous routines / erectile dysfunction in men and loss of libido in women

Body Systems Affected: circulatory, musculoskeletal, endocrine

Inhalation Effect: wakes up the mind and the body, providing a boost of energy to finish the work day or stay awake during classes / shown to be helpful for smokers who want to quit the habit (inhaled when cravings surface)

Dermal Effect: stimulates circulation and warms the body / stimulates the adrenals / helpful for aches and pains at the end of the day / increases blood flow and helpful for male impotence and low sexual drive in women / strengthens orgasmic response in both sexes

Practical Uses: a couple of drops applied neat to the soles of the feet will warm the body during cold, winter months

Vibrational Influence: holds the energy of stamina, ambition and fortitude

Emotional Influence: encourages self-preservation and survival / helps one to dig down deeply to find inner resources when faced with adversity

Synergistic to: nutmeg, basil, juniper berry, ginger

Chakra Correspondence: root, sacral/navel, solar plexus

Cosmetic Use: used in perfumery

Source and Parts Used: dried, unripe fruit of the vine

Caution: *Black pepper is an adrenal stimulant, and individuals with Chronic Fatigue Syndrome, adrenal insufficiency or related disorders should use black pepper sparingly or not at all dermally to avoid further depletion of the adrenal glands. In addition, extreme caution is recommended for those with sensitive kidneys/bladder or kidney disease.*

Bois de Rose See Rosewood

Cacao (Theobroma cacao)

Scent: chocolate, nutty, warm, sweet

Clinical Uses: depression / anxiety / addiction and cravings / neurotransmitter stimulation (serotonin and dopamine) / premenstrual syndrome / sexual apathy or anxiety

Body Systems Affected: nervous/limbic brain

Inhalation Effect: elevates mood / eases sugar and chocolate cravings / calms PMS emotional discomfort / promotes feelings of well-being and joy / inspires creativity / reduces physiological and emotional need to consume comfort foods

Dermal Effect: enhances sensuality and sexual intimacy by releasing endorphins

Practical Uses: great pick-me-up during afternoon slumps or on rainy days / great oil to inhale when attempting to stop smoking or embarking on a path of sobriety or healthier lifestyle

Vibrational Influence: helps transform fear into trusting in a Higher Power and personal, inner strength reserves

Emotional Influence: promotes self-love and forgiveness

Synergistic to: sweet orange, rose, aniseed

Chakra Correspondence: heart, sacral/navel

Cosmetic Use: gorgeous addition to body scrubs, unscented lotion, and facial masks to tighten pores and uplift the spirit / a delicious middle-top note in perfumery

Source and Parts Used: beans from the cacao tree

Caution: *Individuals who are sensitive to caffeine or chocolate should use cacao essential oil a little at a time to see if it's tolerated well. If palpitations and other symptoms are experienced, decrease dose or avoid this essential oil.*

Cajeput (Melaleuca leucadendron)

Scent: similar to eucalyptus with fruity undertones

Clinical Uses: respiratory infections / urinary tract infections / cholera / gout / muscle stiffness / sore throat / pain relief / sciatica / earache

Body Systems Affected: respiratory, urinary, gastrointestinal, musculo-skeletal

Inhalation Effect: opens sinuses and improves breathing

Dermal Effect: boosts immunity / helps clear urinary tract infections / combats cholera

Practical Uses: N/A

Vibrational Influence: offers new perspective and wakes up the spirit

Emotional Influence: brightens outlook

Synergistic to: marjoram, helichrysum

Chakra Correspondence: navel/sacral, heart, throat, brow

Cosmetic Use: used in soaps

Source and Parts Used: leaves and twigs from the tree

Tip: *Be sure to purchase genuine cajeput, for many products labeled as such are synthetic, caustic to the skin, and have no therapeutic value.*

<u>Calendula (Calendula officinalis)</u>

Scent: pungent and musty like marigolds

Clinical Uses: chronic skin conditions / wound care and burns / hair loss from systemic inflammation / burns from radiation therapy

Body Systems Affected: dermal

Inhalation Effect: N/A due to the oil's pungent aroma

Dermal Effect: decreases free radicals that contribute to premature signs of aging / valuable oil for the healing of wounds and burns of all kinds and can be applied neat / reduces systemic inflammation that could lead to some types of hair loss / highly effective for the healing of burns caused by radiation therapy for cancer

Practical Uses: excellent First-Aid essential oil that can be diluted and added to distilled water and sprayed onto wounds or a drop or two applied neat to the area

Vibrational Influence: N/A

Emotional Influence: N/A

Synergistic to: lavender, German chamomile, carrot seed, rose hip

Chakra Correspondence: N/A

Cosmetic Use: used in lotions, cleansers, and anti-aging skin formulas / used in wound-care applications

Source and Parts Used: flowers of the marigold plant

Tip: Until recently, calendula was only available as an *infused oil* (enfleurage or maceration process) not a true essential oil. If you purchase calendula essential oil, be sure it is *true essential oil from the distilled flowers*

Caraway Seed (Carum carvi)

Scent: brightly pungent with peppery undertones

Clinical Uses: nervous indigestion / children's colic / colds / bronchitis

Body Systems Affected: gastrointestinal, respiratory

Inhalation Effect: reduces mental and emotional fatigue

Dermal Effect: calms griping of the intestines, flatulence, and indigestion / breaks up coughs

Practical Uses: N/A

Vibrational Influence: brightens energy field of people and places

Emotional Influence: clears confusion and brings clarity

Synergistic to: anise seed, coriander, cardamom

Chakra Correspondence: sacral/navel, solar plexus, heart

Cosmetic Use: added to soaps and shampoos for skin and scalp problems

Source and Parts Used: seeds and sometimes leaves of the aromatic plant

Cardamom (Elettaria cardamomum)

Scent: spicy, pungent

Clinical Uses: indigestion / poor appetite / nausea / IBS symptoms / colitis / nervous exhaustion / tension / stomach and intestinal spasms / sciatica / nausea from chemotherapy

Body Systems Affected: gastrointestinal, nervous, immune

Inhalation Effect: calms worried minds / eases coughs, breaks up sinus and lung congestion / may ease morning sickness / helpful for nausea from chemotherapy / may help balance the mood and prevent mood swings

Dermal Effect: calms nerves / soothes stomach and intestinal cramping / aids digestion / helpful for nausea from chemotherapy when diluted and applied to the stomach; for best results use in combination with inhalation

Practical Uses: antiseptic for household cleaning / **Tip:** Cardamom will neutralize the odor of garlic on skin or countertops

Vibrational Influence: helps one to remain stable and logical during times of worry and tension / opens the heart to receive more passion and pleasure in everyday life

Synergistic to: ginger

Emotional Influence: eases worry and anxiety

Chakra Correspondence: root, sacral/navel, solar plexus, heart

Cosmetic Use: adds a spicy middle note to perfumes—a drop goes a long way

Source and Parts Used: seeds from the aromatic spice plant

Carrot Seed (Daucus carota)

Scent: earthy-sweet

Clinical Uses: detoxification / congested liver / healing of wounds, burns, and scars / osteoarthritis / cleanses kidneys / helps regulate menstruation / lowers "bad" cholesterol / sluggish elimination / constipation

Body Systems Affected: dermal, endocrine, musculoskeletal, reproductive

Inhalation Effect: imparts a sense of wellbeing, safety, and stability

Dermal Effect: encourages new skin cells and skin rejuvenation / protects skins from UV rays / may prevent skin cancers / supports liver function

Practical Uses: a natural sunscreen when small amount (1-2 drops) is added to moisturizer or lotion

Vibrational Influence: from an Eastern perspective, helps dissolve emotions stored in the tissues, especially anger stored in the liver and fear

in the kidneys / gently assists healing of childhood traumas / can be used in vision quests

Emotional Influence: calms a quick temper, soothes the pain of loneliness

Synergistic to: rose hip seed, rose, lavender, helichrysum

Chakra Correspondence: navel/sacral, solar plexus

Cosmetic Use: excellent for skin health at any age / aids in healing of scars / adds a unique middle note to perfumes / especially soothing to the skin when combined with lavender, rose hip, or rose absolute

Source and Parts Used: seed from the plant also known as Queen Ann's lace

Caution: *Individuals on blood thinners should avoid dermal use of carrot seed/root essential oil. According to some sources, epileptics and anyone prone to seizures should avoid using carrot seed or carrot root essential oil.*

Tip: For high-quality, authentic product, look for oil that is a deep, golden color. This rather expensive oil can be purchased in affordable diluted form and possesses the same properties and scent.

<u>Cassia Bark</u> (Cinnamomum cassia)

a.k.a. cassia cinnamon and Chinese Cinnamon

Scent: sweet and spicy, similar to cinnamon bark

Clinical Uses: indigestion, nausea, diarrhea / serious and stubborn infections including typhoid / fatigue, mental dullness / low libido / uterine hemorrhaging / vascular disorders / melancholy

Body Systems Affected: immune, reproductive, circulatory, nervous

Inhalation Effect: *Direct inhalation is not recommended,* for cassia can severely burn the nasal passages and eyes. Non-direct inhalation (via diffuser for very short periods of time and in an area where it will not be close to eyes and nasal passages, children, and pets) can increase physical energy and mental alertness, improve mood, and stimulate sexual response

Dermal Effect: _Cassia can only be safely applied to the soles of the feet—_ 2 drops per foot is recommended for cases of infectious conditions; for sensitive individuals, use 1 drop or dilute in ¼ teaspoon of carrier oil and then apply to soles of the feet; effective for stubborn bacterial or viral infections when used properly and safely

Practical Uses: will kill bacteria and viruses in the air when used safely in diffuser / nice oil to scent the home, especially in potpourri or sachets / can be rubbed onto candles with a cotton swab for a lovely scent; wait at least 4 hours before burning

Vibrational Influence: fills energy field with positive energy and the spirit of victory / aligns the psyche with abundance, prosperity, and passionate expression

Emotional Influence: lifts the spirit / instills ambition and hope / inspires a sense of security and sense of "home"

Synergistic to: clove, white thyme

Chakra Correspondence: root, navel/sacral, heart

Cosmetic Use: N/A except small amounts can be used as a natural perfume when combined with balsam fir or ylang ylang and dabbed onto the hair (_not_ the scalp)

Source and Parts Used: bark from the tree

Caution: _Cassia should never be applied directly to the skin other than the soles of the feet; serious burns and irritation can result. Individuals on blood thinners should avoid dermal use of cassia essential oil._

Cedar, Atlas* (Cedrus atlantica)

Scent: musty evergreen with subtle spicy undertones

Clinical Uses: chronic and acute anxiety/ urinary complaints including cystitis / alopecia / insomnia / arteriosclerosis / ADHD / scalp disorders / bronchitis / Alzheimer's disease / melatonin production

Body Systems Affected: nervous/limbic, urinary, circulatory, respiratory

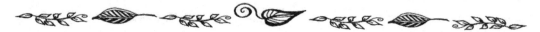

Inhalation Effect: regulates stress hormones / induces sleep by stimulating melatonin production / may promote grounding and centeredness in cases of ADD and ADHD / helps break up lung congestion

Dermal Effect: promotes sleep / calms stressed nervous system / beneficial for alopecia and scalp conditions when massaged into scalp / promotes healing of bronchitis when diluted and rubbed onto the chest or applied neat to the soles of the feet

Practical Uses: N/A

Vibrational Influence: protects the energy field from draining outside influences / raises one's frequency / wonderful oil to add to meditation blends

Emotional Influence: provides a sense of well-being and trust in the outcome / regulates stress hormones and the fight or flight response

Synergistic to: sandalwood, amrys, frankincense, balsam fir, black spruce, pine

Chakra Correspondence: root, heart, solar plexus, brow, crown

Cosmetic Use: a hint to soaps or perfumes for an earthy component

Source and Parts Used: wood from the tree

Tip: Atlas cedar is the only true cedarwood essential oil. Essential oils extracted from species of juniper shrubs are often sold as cedarwood or Texas cedarwood and do not have the same properties as Atlas cedar. Atlas cedar is a descendant of the famed ancient cedars of Lebanon (*Cedrus libani*) and is considered to have been the first extracted essential oil. The aroma of Atlas cedar deepens and mellows nicely with age.

Cedar, Texas (Juniperus virginiana & Juniperus mexicana)

Scent: typical scent of cedar chests

Clinical Uses: diuretic / scalp conditions / alopecia / lung congestion / nervous tension

Body Systems Affected: urinary, nervous, dermal, respiratory

Inhalation Effect: improves breathing and decongests the head and lungs / calms nerves

Dermal Effect: a small amount diluted and combined with pine needle or juniper berry essential oil makes a fragrant and effective chest rub for colds and flu / decreases water retention and stimulates urine production

Practical Uses: Texas cedar keeps away moths and other pests / makes a delightful and economical air freshener or room spray / nice scent to use for clothes when sprinkled generously onto a damp wash cloth and added with wet clothes in the dryer

Vibrational Influence: clears people and places of negativity

Emotional Influence: inspires fortitude

Synergistic to: juniper berry

Chakra Correspondence: root, solar plexus

Cosmetic Use: used in perfumery

Source and Parts Used: wood from the tree

Tip: Do not confuse Texas Cedar with Atlas cedar. Texas cedar is not true cedar and possesses completely different properties. When "cedar" is listed in reliable aromatherapy texts, it always refers to Atlas cedar unless noted. Professional practitioners often see Atlas cedar as the only cedar worth mentioning for clinical applications.

Celery Seed (Apium graveolens)

Scent: herbaceous with spicy, green, and musty undertones

Clinical Uses: liver detoxification and protection / gout and reduction of uric acid / diuretic / osteoarthritis / hepatitis / lactation / nervous disorders / neuralgia / sluggish lymphatic system / rheumatism / cellulite / sciatica / indigestion / weak appetite / diabetes

Body Systems Affected: urinary, gastrointestinal, musculoskeletal, endocrine, nervous, circulatory

Inhalation Effect: calming, good before sleep

Dermal Effect: beneficial for sciatic pain when diluted and rubbed onto lower back and buttocks / calms gastrointestinal complaints when diluted and rubbed onto belly / good addition to anxiety formulas / may be useful for non-insulin-dependent diabetics to lower blood sugar

Practical Uses: disinfectant

Vibrational Influence: eases anxiety and helps one process anger

Emotional Influence: encourages inner peace and willpower when undertaking more positive habits and lifestyle choices

Synergistic to: carrot seed, lemon, sweet fennel, geranium

Chakra Correspondence: solar plexus, root

Cosmetic Use: improves appearance of cellulite / fragrance for soaps

Source and Parts Used: seeds from the celery plant

Chamomile, German (Matricaria recutita)

a.k.a. Blue Chamomile

Scent: woody and floral with honey-like undertones

Clinical Uses: general systemic inflammation / migraine / menstrual pain / nervous disorders / burns and skin problems / indigestion / nausea / nervous bowel / colic / cystitis / joint inflammation and pain / eczema and dermatitis / liver and gall bladder support / female complaints including painful menstruation / carpal tunnel syndrome / nausea from chemotherapy / neurotransmitter imbalances that cause mental illness

Body Systems Affected: gastrointestinal, dermal, reproductive, nervous, muscular, endocrine

Inhalation Effect: acts as an antispasmodic / calms fight or flight response / reduces anxiety and panic / helps to ease tendency to worry

Dermal Effect: soothes and helps to heal burns, sunburn and irritated skin / calms nervous belly and symptoms of Irritable Bowel Syndrome when diluted and rubbed onto the abdomen / calms an overwrought nervous system diluted and applied along the spine / promotes bile production /

antispasmodic for muscles / helps ease menstrual pain, and tones the female reproductive system / helps to break up scar tissue / may be beneficial for carpal tunnel syndrome when diluted and applied to forearm, shoulder, and neck / can be diluted and applied to abdomen and lower back for nausea from chemotherapy / may be helpful for mental illness and chemical-neurotransmitter imbalances that tend to result in extreme moods that swing from high to low

Practical Uses: excellent oil to promote healing of cuts, burns, rashes, and wounds

Vibrational Influence: beneficial during times of loss, grief, and disappointment

Emotional Influence: calming, nourishing, grounding / beneficial after the death of a loved one or the ending of a relationship / dissipates feelings of anger, especially unresolved emotions from past experiences

Synergistic to: Roman chamomile, blue yarrow, helichrysum, rosewood, lavender, neroli, ylang ylang, geranium

Chakra Correspondence: root, sacral/navel, solar plexus, heart

Cosmetic Use: soothes dry and sensitive skin / ingredient in lotions and balms

Source and Parts Used: flowers and buds from the plant

Caution: *Individuals on blood thinners should avoid dermal use of German chamomile essential oil.*

Tip: German chamomile is one of the few essential oils to possess a true blue, greenish-blue, or blue-black color. It is considered to have a stronger effect than Roman chamomile. This rather expensive oil can be purchased in affordable diluted form and possesses the same properties and scent.

Please note that products with the name <u>Wild Chamomile</u> are not from true chamomile and do not possess the same soothing properties; on the contrary, Wild Chamomile is a stimulant.

Chamomile, Roman (Chamaemelum nobile)

Scent: fruity (apple-like), herbaceous and bright

Clinical Uses: indigestion / nervous stomach, morning sickness / anxiety and melancholy / symptoms of mild to moderate depression / skin disorders / menstrual discomfort / children's distress / toothache / nerve regeneration and fortification / blood detoxification / ADHD / eating disorders especially anorexia nervosa / water retention / seasonal allergies and hay fever (only for individuals not sensitive or allergic to ragweed) / chemical imbalances of the nervous system

Body Systems Affected: gastrointestinal, reproductive, nervous/limbic, circulatory, endocrine, dermal, urinary

Inhalation Effect: elevates mood / stimulates healthy appetite / calms worries and anxiety / releases endorphins in the brain that can decrease or eradicate phobias, anxiety, and psychological issues related to eating and food / may be helpful for mental illness and neurotransmitter imbalances

Dermal Effect: helps to heal burns and irritated skin / improves liver function which may improve skin health / cleanses the blood / may assist in weight loss / soothes menstrual cramps when diluted and massaged on abdomen and lower back

Practical Uses: soothes the pain of burns, cuts, and sunburn / disinfectant

Vibrational Influence: assists in the healing of childhood emotional wounds / helps align the energy field with the healing aspects of nature and the Devic kingdom / cleanses the energy field

Emotional Influence: inspires hope / helps one process pain from the past/ beneficial during times of deep disappointment

Synergistic to: German chamomile, coriander seed, rose, lavender

Chakra Correspondence: sacral/navel, solar plexus, heart, brow

Cosmetic Use: lotions and balms for sensitive skin / gives sheen to the hair when added to shampoo or final rinse

Source and Parts Used: flowers from the aromatic plant

Caution: *Individuals on blood thinners should avoid dermal use of Roman chamomile. Roman chamomile should be not be used by individuals who*

are allergic to the plant family of asteraceae compositae family which includes ragweed, marigolds, daisies, and asters/chrysanthemums.

Tip: *Roman chamomile shares the same properties of German or blue chamomile but is gentler and especially recommended for children. This rather expensive oil can be purchased in affordable diluted form and possesses the same properties and scent.

Please note that products labeled as <u>Wild Chamomile</u> *are not true chamomile and do not possess the same soothing properties; on the contrary, wild chamomile is a stimulant.*

<u>Cinnamon Bark</u> (Cinnamomum zeylanicum)

Scent: sweet, warm, and pungent

Clinical Uses: acute conditions such as viral and bacterial infections including typhoid and herpes / warts / parasites / candida overgrowth in the gut / serious tropical infections

Body Systems Affected: immune, gastrointestinal

Inhalation Effect: *cinnamon can irritate the mucus membranes, so please do not inhale directly.* When diffused into the air via nebulizer, cinnamon will kill bacteria, molds, and viruses upon contact / highly effective for sick rooms / uplifts the spirit and wakes up the body and mind on sluggish days when added to potpourri to scent the room / Tip: cassia is a great substitute for more expensive cinnamon for scenting the home or office

Dermal Effect: 1 drop diluted in a carrier oil can be applied to the *soles of the feet only* for a powerful immune booster in cases of serious and acute infection, candida overgrowth, or parasites / a speck of cinnamon oil applied to a wart with a toothpick a few times a week is an excellent remedy (be sure not to apply to the surrounding skin)

Practical Uses: powerfully effective air freshener when added to spray blends for the kitchen or the bathroom

Vibrational Influence: attracts opportunity, success, and abundance

Emotional Influence: instills confidence, mental stamina, hope, and passion

Synergistic to: clove, ginger, oregano

Chakra Correspondence: root, sacral/navel

Cosmetic Use: *N/A except for a drop or two in perfumes that will not touch the skin (applied to the hair only); wart eliminator (see dermal effect)*

Source and Parts Used: wood from the tree

Caution: *Individuals on blood thinners should avoid dermal use of cinnamon bark essential oil. Cinnamon bark essential oil can cause serious burns and skin irritation when used improperly- please take the warnings seriously and never apply undiluted to any part of the body except the soles of the feet or diluted and applied to the soles of the feet. Avoid contact with mucus membranes including eyes, nose, and mouth as well as the genital area. Vapors should not some too close to the eyes or nose, for they can cause irritation. Do not use on children and do not diffuse into the air via nebulizer around children under 5 years of age.*

<u>Cinnamon Leaf</u> (Cinnamomum zeylanicum)

Scent: Spicy, sweet, and bright with subtle minty undertones

Clinical Uses: bronchial conditions / melancholy / morning or afternoon tiredness or sluggishness / bacterial and viral infections

Body Systems Affected: respiratory, immune, brain/limbic, gastrointestinal, musculoskeletal

Inhalation Effect: lifts melancholy, boredom, and apathy / helps reduce sinus inflammation (*to avoid mucus membrane irritation, only use in a diffuser, rather than a steam*) <u>Caution</u>: *Avoid coming in contact with eyes.*

Dermal Effect: soothes digestive spasms when a drop or two is added to a lotion and applied to the abdominal area / decreases muscle aches and pains, especially those associated with influenza / soothes menstrual cramps when diluted and applied to lower back and lower abdominal area

Practical Uses: excellent air freshener when used in room sprays and disinfecting agent for countertop cleaners

Vibrational Influence: helps to clear obsessive thoughts and emotional, psychic, and spiritual attachments that are not beneficial to the individual / cleanses the energy field

Emotional Influence: uplifts the spirit and inspires hope / helps emotional exhaustion

Synergistic to: clove, wintergreen, bay (Pimenta racemosa)

Chakra Correspondence: heart, brow, crown

Cosmetic Use: miniscule amount in perfume blends and soaps, a little goes a long way

Source and Parts Used: leaves from the tree

Caution: *Individuals on blood thinners should avoid cinnamon leaf essential oil. Do not use on children.*

Cistus (Cistus landaniferus)
a.k.a. Rock Rose, Rose of Sharon, and Labdanum

Scent: musky-sweet and resinous

Clinical Uses: multiple sclerosis / dysentery/diarrhea / suppressed menstruation / cell regeneration / slow-healing and infected wounds / skin ulcers / chronic rhinitis / spinal degeneration

Body Systems Affected: nervous, dermal, gastrointestinal, reproductive, respiratory

Inhalation Effect: helps stop chronic sinus drip / uplifts mood

Dermal Effect: has a positive effect on the nervous system / helps resolve serious intestinal conditions such as dysentery / can be applied to wounds to speed healing / promotes menstruation / excellent for toning mature skin / helpful for spinal degeneration when used in massage and applied along the spine

Practical Uses: N/A

Vibrational Influence: elevates vibrational levels of the body

Emotional Influence: improves the mood

Synergistic to: frankincense, sandalwood, lavender

Chakra Correspondence: root, sacral/navel

Cosmetic Use: added to cosmetics and used to firm tired skin

Source and Parts Used: leaves of the flowering shrub

<u>Clary Sage</u> (Salvia sclarea)

Scent: grassy, herbaceous, green

Clinical Uses: female hormone balance / menopausal discomforts such as hot flashes and night sweats / neurotransmitter production (dopamine) / mild to moderate symptoms of depression including post-partum / anxiety and panic attacks / blood sugar balance / stressed adrenals / sluggish kidneys / food and substance cravings, substance withdrawal / debility / cholesterol balance

Body Systems Affected: endocrine, nervous system/limbic brain, reproductive

Inhalation Effect: uplifts mood and helps to even out mood swings / inspires confidence / stimulates the production of dopamine / may be useful for cravings and withdrawal / shown to be helpful for smokers who want to quit the habit (inhaled when cravings surface) especially when combined with bergamot / may help women achieve orgasm more easily

Dermal Effect: balances blood sugar in individuals prone to high blood sugar / may help to lower high cholesterol / balances estrogen and progesterone especially beneficial during times of PMS and menopause / calms the nervous system / has estrogen-like effect on the body

Practical Uses: disinfectant

Vibrational Influence: opens the energy field to experiencing joy / tempers tendency to worry and overthink / promotes self-acceptance during changes in life or health

Emotional Influence: instills courage, bravery, and hope during times of transition, new beginnings, or undertakings / helps the emotional self align with the sexual self

Synergistic to: geranium, bergamot, anise, grapefruit, rose

Chakra Correspondence: root, sacral/navel, solar plexus

Cosmetic Use: a drop or two added to lotions can be calming, especially after a stressful day / soothes irritated skin / plumps skin and reduces appearance of wrinkles

Source and Parts Used: flowering tops and leaves of the plant

Caution: *Clary sage is contraindicated in cases of estrogen-dependent cancer and cancer in general. Individuals on blood thinners should avoid dermal use of clary sage essential oil. Clary sage should not be used when a person is or plans to be under the influence of alcohol as it enhances drunkenness due to its capability of stimulating dopamine in the brain. Clary sage should be used in moderation by anyone with reactive/non-diabetic hypoglycemia (low blood sugar.)*

Clove Bud (Syzygium aromaticum)

Scent: pungent, spicy

Clinical Uses: immune-protection during winter months / bacterial, viral, and systemic fungal infections / Lyme disease / diarrhea / blood clot prevention / toothache and gingivitis / may be helpful to fight cancer / promoting vivid dreams and recall / poor concentration and memory / fear, anxiety and physical symptoms associated with it / hepatitis B and C / E.coli, Listeria, and Salmonella / head lice / phobias / osteoarthritis / leukemia / bursitis / thyroid imbalance (hyper/hypothyroidism) / chronic viruses and chronic symptoms from viral infections / smoking cessation

Body Systems Affected: immune, endocrine, digestive, nervous, musculoskeletal

Inhalation Effect: sharpens memory, articulation, and dream recall / calms fear, especially useful for phobias and hypochondria / may be helpful for

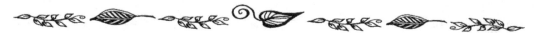

quitting smoking and reducing cravings **Note**: *Be sure to keep away from nasal passages and avoid steam inhalation. Use a drop on a folded tissue instead or in an aroma locket*

Dermal Effect: fights contagious diseases and excellent for any bacterial, viral, or fungal infection including Lyme disease / excellent for halting diarrhea and abdominal pain when diluted and applied to abdomen / for systemic candida overgrowth / lessens muscle and joint pain, and warms soft tissues by improving circulation when added to blends or lotions / decreases inflammation associated with bursitis / helps to balance excessive or too little thyroid hormones / withdraws chronic viruses stuck or dormant in tissues / draws pathogens from the bones

Practical Uses: will prevent and kill head lice / tick repellant / highly-effective oil for household disinfectant

Vibrational Influence: inspires strength and fortitude while calming the nerves / rids the energy field of parasitic psychic energies

Emotional Influence: calms racing thoughts and fears / gives a sense of safety and "roots" during times of transition

Synergistic to: cinnamon, cassia, lemon, white thyme

Chakra Correspondence: root, sacral/navel, heart

Cosmetic Use: adds spicy overtones to perfumes and soaps (small amounts and diluted properly)

Source and Parts Used: from the flowering buds of the tree

Caution: *Be careful using clove essential oil if taking medications such as Warfarin, aspirin, and Coumadin, for clove may affect the prescribed dose of medication. Clove may inhibit bonding during crown procedures and is advised to not use clove oil before getting a crown. Clove essential oil is caustic to the skin, so please dilute well for dermal use (1 drop per teaspoon of carrier oil) unless applying to the soles of the feet.*

Tip: like lavender, lemon, white thyme, and tea tree oil, clove is considered to be a universal oil and rallies against viruses, bacteria, and fungus.

Coffee Bean (Coffea arabica)

Scent: freshly-brewed coffee

Clinical Uses: improvement of memory and brain function / symptoms of mild-moderate depression / dopamine and other neurotransmitter production

Body Systems Affected: nervous/limbic, dermal

Inhalation Effect: may minimize nausea when inhaled / releases dopamine and other endorphins, thus lifting lethargy, boredom, and low moods

Dermal Effect: (see Cosmetic Use)

Practical Uses: may be useful for stings and insect bites

Vibrational Influence: helps one to lift the weight of the past and move forward with hope and resilience

Emotional Influence: instills ambition and readiness to take on tasks at hand

Synergistic to: cacao

Chakra Correspondence: root, solar plexus

Cosmetic Use: useful to plump, tighten, and cleanse the skin / helps reduce appearance of cellulite / adds a luscious middle-top note to perfume blends

Source and Parts Used: beans from the plant

Caution: *It is strongly advised that people who are sensitive to caffeine, have certain heart conditions, reactive/non-diabetic hypoglycemia (low blood sugar), or suffer from anxiety disorders to avoid coffee essential oil entirely to avoid unpleasant reactions.*

Copaiba (Copaifera officinalis)

Scent: mild, sweet, and slightly evergreen

Clinical Uses: stubborn skin conditions / respiratory conditions such as bronchitis / inflammatory conditions, autoimmune disorders / Lupus / fibromyalgia / osteoarthritis and rheumatoid arthritis pain / bladder incontinence / cystitis / diarrhea / herpes / tuberculosis / fungal infections / improvement of heart function and heart health by decreasing PGE2 production / inducing homeostasis of the body

Body Systems Affected: dermal, respiratory, gastrointestinal, musculoskeletal, nervous, circulatory

Inhalation Effect: useful for sinusitis / reduces nervousness / improves quality of breathing

Dermal Effect: lessens inflammatory pain and inflammation in general / excellent for fungal infections and stubborn skin conditions / fortifies the kidneys and bladder, especially when diluted and applied to the kidney area / helpful in preventing and decreasing the duration of herpes outbreaks / a beneficial chest rub for colds, bronchitis, and flu when added to lotion, carrier oil, or aloe vera gel / speeds healing of wounds

Practical Uses: for skin health and healing

Vibrational Influence: similar to the vibrational properties of sandalwood / stills the mind and elevates the spirit

Emotional Influence: comforting, soothing, and helps to balance emotional extremes

Synergistic to: helichrysum, frankincense, myrrh, sandalwood

Chakra Correspondence: all

Cosmetic Use: excellent for wounds, scars, acne, and the healing of skin conditions such as dermatitis. Dilute for sensitive skin.

Source and Parts Used: resin from the tree

Tip: Copaiba is considered to be one of the most powerful substances yet discovered for rallying against inflammation. It is also very useful in veterinary care.

Coriander Seed (Coriandrum sativum)

Scent: musky with subtle spice and licorice-like undertones

Clinical Uses: diabetes / infections / stubborn skin conditions / gout / lung infections / measles / digestive upset and flatulence / weak appetite / nervous exhaustion and debility / menstrual pain / muscle and joint pain / conditions related to low estrogen in women / pancreas support / neuralgia / anorexia nervosa

Body Systems Affected: dermal, endocrine, nervous, respiratory, immune, gastrointestinal, nervous

Inhalation Effect: improves mental function / uplifts the mood yet calms the body / stimulates appetite / supports and strengthens the pancreas / eating disorders

Dermal Effect: useful to balance blood sugar and insulin / calms nervous and upset stomach and intestines when added to carrier oil or lotion and applied to the abdomen / eases coughs and congestion when diluted and rubbed onto chest / lessens pain in soft tissues and pain associated with neuralgia / may be helpful for eating disorders

Practical Uses: used as an analgesic when added to carrier oil

Vibrational Influence: fosters a sense of security

Emotional Influence: instills calm and balance

Synergistic to: anise seed, cardamom, celery seed, dill

Chakra Correspondence: root, sacral/navel, solar plexus

Cosmetic Use: reduces and helps remove blackheads / adds a musky heart note to perfumes (a little goes a long way) / lovely addition to facial toners

Source and Parts Used: seeds from the aromatic plant

Caution: *Individuals with reactive/non-diabetic hypoglycemia (low blood sugar) should use coriander seed essential oil sparingly. Diabetics should be cautious when using coriander, for the need for insulin may be affected in terms of dose.*

Cumin (Cuminum cyminum)

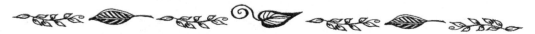

Scent: extremely pungent, earthy with spicy undertones

Clinical Uses: toxic liver / malignancies / digestive sluggishness / cholera / diarrhea / scanty urine / hyperthyroidism

Body Systems Affected: digestive, endocrine

Inhalation Effect: may alleviate headaches when used in small amounts for brief periods of time

Dermal Effect: due to its pungent odor, it is not the first oil of choice to use for certain conditions, but small amounts can be diluted and rubbed on the abdomen in cases of cholera, diarrhea, or compromised liver function / balances excessive thyroid hormone production

Practical Uses: N/A

Vibrational Influence: protects people and places from malevolent energies

Emotional Influence: uplifts the mood if aroma is pleasant to the individual

Synergistic to: coriander, cardamom, angelica

Chakra Correspondence: root, sacral/navel, solar plexus

Cosmetic Use: miniscule amounts in perfumery

Source and Parts Used: seeds from the aromatic plant

Cypress (Cupressus sempervirens)

Scent: pungently woody and cedar-like

Clinical Uses: sluggish circulation / varicose veins / hemorrhoids / excessive menstrual bleeding and cramps / lymphatic congestion / edema / asthma and bronchial spasms / benign cysts / muscle pain and stiffness / systemic congestion / angina / asthma / acute grief when the body is affected by loss or shock / connective tissue support

Body Systems Affected: circulatory, lymphatic, respiratory, musculo-skeletal

Inhalation Effect: helps reduce sinus congestion / instills emotional equilibrium during and after the death of a loved one

Dermal Effect: excellent to improve blood and lymphatic circulation / tones the veins of the body / relieves chest congestion and respiratory spasms / helpful to reduce asthma attacks when diluted and rubbed onto the chest and throat / helps to detoxify lymphatic system / strengthens capillaries and connective tissue / eases muscle and joint pain and brings pleasant, warming relief to affected areas / helps to ease menstrual cramping when added to bath water, or diluted and applied to the abdomen and lower back

Practical Uses: excellent oil to apply, especially with peppermint, to the soles of the feet when traveling to avoid edema / insect repellant

Vibrational Influence: helps an individual to weather life's changes and transitions / instills fortitude and multi-level resilience

Emotional Influence: helps one through the process of grief or one's own process of dying—not only physical death but also the death of relationships, long-held hopes or dreams, or any other transition involving loss and transformation / encourages the willingness to survive

Synergistic to: myrrh, pine, black spruce, frankincense, sandalwood

Chakra Correspondence: root, heart, crown

Cosmetic Use: Added in small amounts to perfumes for a deep, earthy quality.

Source and Parts Used: needles and twigs of the tree

Cypress, Australian Blue (Callitris intratropica)

Scent: pleasantly woody with sweet evergreen overtones

Clinical Uses: herpes simplex and herpes zoster / viral infections / lung and breath support / overall immune strengthening

Body Systems Affected: immune, respiratory

Inhalation Effect: uplifts the spirit and soothes agitation / calms without sedating

Dermal Effect: fights herpes flare-ups including cold sores / wards off viruses / apply neat to the soles of the feet and used diluted in massage

Practical Uses: insect repellant

Vibrational Influence: instills grounding and practicality with a sense of joy

Emotional Influence: inspires happiness, hope, and contentment

Synergistic to: sandalwood, German chamomile

Chakra Correspondence: root, solar plexus

Cosmetic Use: moisturizer for dry skin and skin exposed to hot climates

Source and Parts Used: bark, heartwood, and sapwood of the tree

<u>Davana</u> (Artemisia pallens)

Scent: pleasantly complex and fruity

Clinical Uses: high blood pressure / tetanus and wounds / low libido / headaches of nervous origin / for mild-moderate depression / melancholy

Body Systems Affected: immune, nervous/limbic

Inhalation Effect: calms frayed nerves / helps the body to feel more pleasure / heightens the senses / brightens the spirits

Dermal Effect: antimicrobial and helps wounds to heal

Practical Uses: excellent deodorant when diluted and applied to skin

Vibrational Influence: helps the spirit to align with joy, peace, and aesthetic beauty

Emotional Influence: inspires being in the moment / instills joy and hope

Synergistic to: ylang ylang, bergamot, clary sage

Chakra Correspondence: root, sacral/navel, solar plexus, heart, crown

Cosmetic Use: used in perfumery, soaps, and deodorants / effective for wound care

Source and Parts Used: leaves and flowers of the plant

Dill (Anethum graveolens)

Scent: "green" and herbaceous, pleasantly sharp

Clinical Uses: diabetes / nervousness / nervous stomach and digestive upset / ADHD / food and sugar cravings

Body Systems Affected: gastrointestinal, endocrine, nervous/limbic

Inhalation Effect: may help to reduce sugar and alcohol cravings / calms anxiety and brightens the mood / beneficial for ADHD when diffused into the air with Roman chamomile / improves appetite / balances over-excited autonomic nervous system

Dermal Effect: improves pancreatic function and may be useful for diabetics who want to control their blood sugar levels with less administered insulin / decreases gas in the digestive tract / antispasmodic for digestive spasms and pain

Practical Uses: adds a fragrant antimicrobial and antibacterial agent to kitchen/household cleaners

Vibrational Influence: cleanses heaviness in the energy field / like sunlight in a dark room for the spirit

Emotional Influence: calms worries and scattered thoughts / instils confidence in one's abilities

Synergistic to: coriander, Roman chamomile, celery seed

Chakra Correspondence: solar plexus

Cosmetic Use: soap making

Source and Parts Used: seeds of the fragrant plant

Caution: *Epileptics and anyone prone to seizures should not use dill essential oil. Anyone with reactive/non-diabetic hypoglycemia (low blood sugar) should use dill very sparingly. Diabetics should be cautious using dill as it could affect their required insulin doses.*

Elemi (Canarium luzonicum)

Scent: eucalyptus-like with lemon overtones

Clinical Uses: chest infections / excessive phlegm / chronic bronchitis

Body Systems Affected: respiratory, dermal

Inhalation Effect: relieves sinus congestion and post nasal drip / calms the mind and body

Dermal Effect: combats chest ailments and infections when diluted and rubbed on the chest and throat / moisturizes and enlivens dry and mature skin / reduce scars / minimizes appearance of wrinkles

Practical Uses: sometimes used to flavor foods and beverages / scent in detergents

Vibrational Influence: encourages strength of spirit

Emotional Influence: calms the mind and can be useful prior to meditation

Synergistic to: frankincense, myrrh, Atlas cedarwood

Chakra Correspondence: root, heart, throat, brow, and crown

Cosmetic Use: soothes irritated, dry, mature, or scarred skin / cosmetics and soaps

Source and Parts Used: resin from the tree

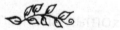

EUCALYPTUS*

*There are over 700 species of eucalyptus trees in the world. Here are a few of the most widely-used in aromatic medicine.

...

Eucalyptus Citriodora a.k.a. Lemon Eucalyptus (*Eucalyptus citriodora*)

Scent: menthol with pungent citrus and citronella overtones

Clinical Uses: colds and flu / viral respiratory infections / bronchitis / shingles / muscle and joint pain / cravings associated with alcohol addiction

Body Systems Affected: respiratory, musculoskeletal, immune

Inhalation Effect: helps to clear up sinusitis and sinus congestion / soothes and speeds healing of head colds / lifts the mood when one has the 'blues' / may be helpful in boosting neurotransmitters, therefore, reducing alcohol cravings

Dermal Effect: when blended with fir or spruce, very effective for muscle and joint pain, especially pain associated with flu and colds / breaks up chest congestion when diluted and applied as a chest rub / helps combat shingles / highly effective for bacterial and viral infections of the respiratory system

Practical Uses: repels mosquitoes, cockroaches, ticks, and silverfish / repels insects when diluted and sprayed on the clothes before a hike or spending time outdoors

Vibrational Influence: helps to foster new beginnings by clearing out the old on the subconscious level / helps one to change consciousness about a situation past or present

Emotional Influence: brightens the mood and invites balance / lessens excessive worry, especially about health-related matters

Synergistic to: eucalyptus globulus, lemon, ravensara, melissa (lemon balm)

Chakra Correspondence: heart, throat, and brow

Cosmetic Use: added to soaps and bath salts for a muscle-relaxing soak

Source and Parts Used: leaves and sometimes twigs of the tree

Caution: *Do not use near the face or on the chest in cases of asthma, for menthol can trigger asthmatic attacks in some individuals.*

Eucalyptus Dives (Eucalyptus dives)

a.k.a. Peppermint Eucalyptus

Scent: soft, woody menthol with minty undertones

Clinical Uses: respiratory ailments and infections / throat ailments / muscle pain

Body Systems Affected: respiratory, immune, musculoskeletal

Inhalation Effect: sinus and chest congestion / hastens recovery from throat infections / wakes up the mind and makes one feel more "awake" during afternoon slumps

Dermal Effect: strengthens immune system / minimizes muscle pain

Practical Uses: a drop or two can be added to aloe vera gel and rubbed on the hands before going out in public during cold and flu season

Vibrational Influence: helps us to be gentle with ourselves

Emotional Influence: lessens stress and pressure

Synergistic to: eucalyptus globulus, lavender

Chakra Correspondence: heart, brow

Cosmetic Use: added to cleansers, soaps, and bath salts

Source and Parts Used: leaves and sometimes twigs of the tree

Caution: *do not use near the face or on the chest in cases of asthma, for menthol can trigger asthmatic attacks in some individuals. Do not use on infants or young children.*

Tip: gentler than other forms of eucalyptus and better for those with somewhat sensitive skin or nasal passages

Eucalyptus a.k.a. Blue Gum (Eucalyptus globulus)

Scent: pungent menthol

Clinical Uses: sinus infections / arthritis / respiratory ailments / systemic candida overgrowth / athlete's foot and other fungal conditions of the feet and nails / head lice / bronchial restriction / Staphylococcus bacteria / soft tissue and joint pain and sprains / arthritic swelling / inflammation / infectious fevers such as malaria and typhoid / cholera

Body Systems Affected: immune, respiratory, musculoskeletal, integumentary

Inhalation Effect: potential to clear up stubborn sinus infections and chronic, severe sinusitis / will act as an antihistamine for seasonal allergies and similar allergic responses

Dermal Effect: eases the pain of muscles, joints, and ligaments from overuse, sprains, influenza, and chronic pain syndromes / strengthens the immune system to fight viruses and bacteria / combats infectious fevers / breaks up chest congestion when diluted and applied to the chest and throat in non-asthmatics / kills fungal infections of the feet rather quickly via footbaths / added to hot steam showers and baths to eliminate toxins through the skin

Practical Uses: kills yeasts and molds; a drop or two added to water for house plants will kill any mold or pest infestation in the soil. Also wonderful for a household cleaner

Vibrational Influence: clears the energy field of guilt, shame, and regret

Emotional Influence: promotes a brighter outlook and fosters self-care/self-love

Synergistic to: white thyme, tea tree, lemon

Chakra Correspondence: root, sacral/navel, heart, brow, and crown

Cosmetic Use: added to soaps and cleansers for a deep clean as well as a healing and germ-fighting agent for acne-prone and oily skin / bath products to soothe aching muscles

Source and Parts Used: leaves and sometimes twigs of the tree

Caution: *do not use near the face or on the chest in cases of asthma, for menthol can trigger asthmatic attacks in some individuals. Avoid the eyes.*

Tip: the most commonly-used eucalyptus oil

Eucalyptus Smithii (Eucalyptus smithii)

Scent: bright menthol

Clinical Uses: respiratory ailments and infections / throat ailments / muscle pain

Body Systems Affected: respiratory, immune, musculoskeletal

Inhalation Effect: sinus and chest congestion / hastens recovery from throat infections

Dermal Effect: strengthens immune system / lessens muscle pain

Practical Uses: due to its gentle yet powerful action, a drop or two can be added to aloe vera gel and rubbed on the hands before going out in public during cold and flu season

Vibrational Influence: like other varieties of eucalyptus, clears the energy field of heaviness from negative memories, regret, and guilt

Emotional Influence: promotes self-care

Synergistic to: white thyme, tea tree, lemon

Chakra Correspondence: heart, brow, crown

Cosmetic Use: cleansers and soaps

Source and Parts Used: leaves and sometimes twigs of the tree

Caution: *do not use near the face or on the chest in cases of asthma, for menthol can trigger asthmatic attacks in some individuals.*

Tip: the mildest of all eucalyptus oils and most suitable for children and those with sensitive skin or adversely affected by strong aromatics

Eucalyptus Radiata (Eucalyptus radiata)

Scent: camphorous and bright

Clinical Uses: sore throat / chest infections / excessive heat in the body due to weather or hormones / for burns and skin irritations / head lice / tuberculosis

Body Systems Affected: respiratory, dermal

Inhalation Effect: steam inhalation for sore throats and sinus pain / congestion / may be helpful for tuberculosis

Dermal Effect: cools the body / speeds healing of sore throats and chest ailments / cleans and helps to heal burns, blisters, and skin irritations / may be helpful for tuberculosis when applied neat to the soles of the feet

Practical Uses: a few drops added to cool water in a spray bottle will cool the body on hot days or during menopausal hot flashes / insect repellant / when combined with bergamot essential oil, will speed healing and duration of cold sores when dabbed onto the spot

Vibrational Influence: clears emotional baggage

Emotional Influence: brings balance and lessens extremes / promotes a more relaxed attitude toward life

Synergistic to: peppermint

Chakra Correspondence: heart, throat, brow

Cosmetic Use: skin care, shampoos

Source and Parts Used: leaves and sometimes twigs of the tree

Caution: *do not use near the face or on the chest in cases of asthma, for menthol can trigger asthmatic attacks in some individuals.*

Fennel, Sweet (Foeniculum vulgare)

Scent: anise or licorice-like with green undertones

Clinical Uses: sluggish or painful digestion / weak intestinal peristalsis / stimulation of lactation and reduction of breast pain from nursing / menstrual cramps / phlegm / nagging, allergy-related post nasal drip and cough / hormonal fluid retention in women / low estrogen in women / clears the body of toxins that can cause sluggishness / weak appetite

Body Systems Affected: hormonal, digestive, respiratory

Inhalation Effect: promotes inner tranquility and brighter outlook

Dermal Effect: stimulates breast milk production in nursing mothers when diluted and applied to the body / helps sore breasts to heal and decreases engorgement / helps belly aches, indigestion, flatulence, belching, and sluggish bowels when diluted and applied to abdomen

Practical Uses: a tiny drop under the tongue will freshen breath and aid digestion / adds a delightful scent to all-purpose cleaning sprays for the kitchen

Vibrational Influence: helps to dissolve old patterns that keep us stuck and inspires creative solutions

Emotional Influence: dissolves fear of failure and inspires clarity and confidence

Synergistic to: geranium, anise seed

Chakra Correspondence: sacral/navel, solar plexus, brow

Cosmetic Use: added to fragrances, toothpastes, and soaps for a pleasant licorice-like scent or flavor

Source and Parts Used: seeds from the aromatic plant

Caution: *Sweet fennel is contraindicated for estrogen-dependent cancers, especially cancer of the breast. Do not use sweet fennel essential oil dermally if you are estrogen-dominant or have had breast cancer or any estrogen-dependent malignancy. Epileptics and people with hypothyroidism (low thyroid) should not use sweet fennel.*

Fir, Balsam (Abies balsamea)

Scent: sweet evergreen, Christmas tree

Clinical Uses: adrenal exhaustion / general fatigue / stress-related ailments / urinary tract infections / excessive cortisol and other stress hormones / depression / lung and sinus congestion / muscular and joint pain / strained muscles / fibromyalgia muscle pain and deep aching /

stimulation of Human Growth Hormone (HGH) / rheumatoid arthritis / osteoarthritis

Body Systems Affected: endocrine, respiratory, urinary, musculoskeletal

Inhalation Effect: eases sinus congestion / diminishes harmful effects of excessive cortisol (stress hormone) production

Dermal Effect: balances cortisol production / increases HGH (human growth hormone) / helps the body renew and rejuvenate itself / increases energy stores / breaks up congestion in the lungs and sinuses / may lessen intensity of influenza and colds / eases muscular pain associated with injury, post-workout discomfort, and chronic pain syndromes such as fibromyalgia / supportive to exhausted adrenals (non-Addison's hypoadrenia) / supports the kidneys and bladder / mild-moderate depression especially stemming from low energy reserves, caregiving, or overwork

Practical Uses: antiseptic in household cleaning / air freshener / nice scent to use for clothes when sprinkled generously onto a damp wash cloth and added with wet clothes in the dryer

Vibrational Influence: good oil to use before spending time with a group of people or to cleanse the field after working with people (excellent for therapists, massage therapists, energy workers, teachers, caregivers, etc.) / nourishes and replenishes kidney-adrenal vitality / cleanses the energy field of negative thought-forms / protects the energy field from unwanted outside influences / grounding to the entire individual on all levels

Emotional Influence: inspires fortitude, hope, security, and contentment / emotional nourishment during times of hopelessness, loss, transition, or uncertainty

Synergistic to: pine needle, black spruce, frankincense, juniper berry

Chakra Correspondence: root, navel/sacral, solar plexus, crown

Cosmetic Use: perfumery for men and women

Source and Parts Used: needles and twigs of the tree

Caution: *some people may experience sensitivity to the sun if the oil is*

used dermally prior to exposure to sunlight and/or tanning beds. Wait 24 hours to be sure.

<u>Fir, White</u> a.k.a. Silver Fir (Abies alba, Abies concolor)

Scent: evergreen, Christmas tree

Clinical Uses: strengthening of immunity / muscle and joint pain, strains and sprains / respiratory ailments / physical, emotional, or mental exhaustion / osteoarthritis

Body Systems Affected: endocrine, immune, musculoskeletal, respiratory, nervous/limbic

Inhalation Effect: lifts depression from mental and emotional exhaustion / breaks up congestion of sinuses and lungs / deepens the breath and opens bronchial passages / refreshes the mind

Dermal Effect: decreases muscle and joint pain, wonderful for sprains and strains, decreases pain intensity of pain syndromes such as fibromyalgia / supports the adrenals and kidneys and helps to restore life force / breaks up coughs when diluted and rubbed onto the chest / restores physical and emotional vitality when added to a hot bath

Practical Uses: makes a beautiful air freshener, air mister, and household cleaner

Vibrational Influence: restores energy reserves and is especially suitable for caregivers, nurses, and holistic practitioners

Emotional Influence: restores hope / promotes self-preservation / brings balance to the emotional body after illness, divorce, break-ups, life changes, transitions, disappointments, and the death of a loved one

Synergistic to: cypress, frankincense, pine needle

Chakra Correspondence: root, navel/sacral, solar plexus, heart

Cosmetic Use: soaps, bath salts, and perfumery

Source and Parts Used: needles and twigs of the tree

Caution: *some people may experience sensitivity to the sun if the oil is*

used prior to exposure to sunlight and/or tanning beds. Wait 24 hours to be sure.

Frankincense (Boswellia carteri)

Scent: resinous, slightly musty with subtle citrus undertones

Clinical Uses: male and female hormone balance / hypoxia (low oxygen in tissues) / research shows promising potential for tumor shrinkage and cancer prevention / certain skin cancers / keloid scars / shingles / anxiety and panic attacks / impaired immunity / stimulation of white blood cells / stimulation of HGH (human growth hormone) / nervous exhaustion during and after prolonged stress / symptoms of mild-moderate depression / phobias and fixations / physical symptoms accompanying acute grief / muscle restriction of the diaphragm and shallow breathing / chronic bronchitis and other lung conditions / Alzheimer's disease / autism

Body Systems Affected: endocrine, immune, nervous/limbic, integumentary, respiratory

Inhalation Effect: increases oxygen to the brain / calms the flight or fight stress response / helps the diaphragm to release core-held tension for a deeper and easier breath / may be very helpful for women in labor / minimizes obsessions / may be helpful for certain types of autism / for grief

Dermal Effect: combined with lavender, may prevent or halt certain skin cancers / reduces keloid scars when applied topically / brings equilibrium to the hormonal system and supports balance of thyroid, adrenal, and reproductive hormones as well as neurotransmitters / highly nourishing to the pituitary and hypothalamus which govern hormonal levels in the body / calms an over-excited or hair-trigger autonomic nervous system, especially when diluted and applied along the spine / balances adrenalin / halts panic attacks and anxiety, especially when blended with ylang ylang and lavender and applied along the spine / increases oxygen to the tissues and organs / may be very helpful to women in labor when applied neat to the soles of the feet and diluted and applied to lower back / may be helpful for certain types of autism when applied neat to the soles of the feet

Practical Uses: N/A

Vibrational Influence: strengthens the energy field / integrates emotions and thoughts into a state of unity and acceptance / aligns the self to its highest good / invites spiritual and psychic protection

Emotional Influence: calms the flight or fight response / soothes and may prevent anxiety and panic / promotes inner peace and inspires mental stillness / minimizes obsessions and obsessive thoughts

Synergistic to: sandalwood, myrrh, Atlas cedarwood, spikenard, vetiver

Chakra Correspondence: all

Cosmetic Use: makes dry or mature skin more supple and youthful / apply daily to keloid scars to diminish them

Source and Parts Used: resin from the tree

Tip: For stimulating the parasympathetic nervous system, frankincense may be blended with lavender, ylang ylang, spikenard, and Atlas cedarwood. It is an oil that works best when used consistently over a period of time.

Notes: Frankincense is one of the most important essential oils in modern clinical aromatherapy. Today, according to European studies, frankincense is showing significant promise in the shrinkage of tumors. Clinically, frankincense is a "master" oil as it tends to balance the endocrine system as a whole. Frankincense can be a powerful ally in the area of anxiety and panic disorders. Frankincense may be extremely helpful in changing deep cellular patterns of the body, thus beneficial for adrenal, thyroid, and pituitary function, all which are critical for well-being.

Galbanum (Ferula gummosa)

Scent: pungently bitter, resinous

Clinical Uses: nervousness / intestinal health / inflamed skin conditions / diuretic

Body Systems Affected: dermal, gastrointestinal, urinary, nervous

Inhalation Effect: calms nerves, though the pungency of this oil is not one that is considered pleasant

Dermal Effect: reduces scar tissue / reduces spasms of smooth muscle / diluted and combined with frankincense, helps to reduce appearance of scars / speeds healing of wounds and inflamed skin disorders including abscesses and acne

Practical Uses: acts as a preservative

Vibrational Influence: encourages acceptance and prompts us to see the truth, even in its most unpleasant forms

Emotional Influence: fosters calm focus

Synergistic to: myrrh, frankincense, sandalwood

Chakra Correspondence: root, sacral/navel, crown

Cosmetic Use: reduces appearance of wrinkles / reduces scar tissue / used in small amounts as a fixative in perfumery

Source and Parts Used: resin from the perennial shrub

Geranium (Pelargonium graveolens)

Scent: like the scented leaves of the plant with citrus and rose undertones

Clinical Uses: women's hormonal balance / excessive menstrual bleeding / symptoms of menopause and PMS / balancing liver function / pain associated with shingles / neuralgia / sensitive and irritated skin / tonsillitis / systemic candida / fungal skin infections / gastrointestinal distress, especially from hormone shifts and stress / post-partum depression / adrenal support / homeostasis (harmonious balance of bodily functions and systems) / MRSA / violent emotional swings / acute and suppressed grief

Body Systems Affected: hormonal, endocrine, nervous, integumentary, lymphatic

Inhalation Effect: comforts and soothes the nerves, especially during times of grief, heartache, loss, and transition / eases depression, especially when attributed to fluctuating hormones / calms emotional swings,

especially violent tendencies due to hormone or chemical (neurotransmitter) imbalance

Dermal Effect: helps to heal rashes including chicken pox and shingles / helps heal burns, cuts and scrapes / fungal infections of the skin / decreases and balances systemic yeast overgrowth / helps to heal psoriasis / soothes intestinal upset / supports harmony of the menstrual cycle / combined with lemongrass it is a powerful anti-candida agent / supports the adrenals during times of stress and has adaptogenic qualities, therefore capable of providing calming or gently stimulating effects as we need them / may help to prevent herpes-related outbreaks, including shingles / minimizes broken capillaries on the face / reduces stretch marks

Practical Uses: 1 drop added to water given to house plants will eradicate fungus and molds in the soil (use for a month); for a more powerful mixture, add 2 drops of tea tree oil / makes a wonderful household cleaner when added to distilled water / tick repellant / acts as a gentle and fragrant deodorant

Vibrational Influence: promotes a more yielding nature during times of transition / encourages self-forgiveness, self-preservation, and self-care

Emotional Influence: calms and balances emotional extremes / promotes self-love and helps one to resolve past traumas lodged in the body and the psyche / the primary oil to use during acute grief and emotional shock / possesses energy of the Sacred Feminine / especially helpful for women's grief after the death of a parent or parental figure / uplifts the mind and eases symptoms of depression / inspires hope / helpful for integrating and processing childhood abuse

Synergistic to: clary sage, lemongrass, lavender, clove, bergamot, rose

Chakra Correspondence: root, sacral/navel, heart

Cosmetic Use: reduces stretch marks / excellent when diluted and combined with rosewood, ravensara, frankincense and lavender to lessen duration and pain of shingles rash / excellent for balancing oily skin / 2 drops added to eight ounces of distilled water or pure culinary rose water in a spritzer bottle makes a lovely facial spray and can be used after cleansing, before applying make-up, or as a cool-down method on hot, humid days / can be used as a fragrant deodorant

Source and Parts Used: leaves, stems, and flowers of the aromatic plant

Tip: Geranium essential oil ages beautifully, getting sweeter, deeper and more complex with time.

Notes: While geranium essential oil is highly useful to ease acute or new grief, it may bring up old losses and emotions stored in the body. It is a gentle oil that helps us to grieve when the time is right for us and allows us to face our feelings with a sense of security. ***Note to massage therapists:*** if grief comes up during a session, geranium and rosewood are wonderful oils to reach for to use on a client; apply to the area of the heart chakra and the palms of the hands. If you are using geranium essential oil on a client and grief unexpectedly comes to the surface, stabilizing oils like vetiver, patchouli, or sandalwood are good choices to bring into the session, especially applied neat to the feet.

<u>Geranium, Rose</u> (Pelargonium roseum)

*Note: *Rose geranium essential oil shares the same properties as Geranium (Pelargonium graveolens) but is especially recommended for adrenal fatigue, emotional weariness, and healing and strengthening of the heart center (chakra.)*

Scent: geranium flowers with strong rose undertones, pleasantly sweet; sweeter and more rose-like than common geranium (Pelargonium graveolens)

Clinical Uses: see **Geranium** (Pelargonium graveolens)

Body Systems Affected: see Geranium (Pelargonium graveolens)

Inhalation Effect: see Geranium (Pelargonium graveolens)

Dermal Effect: see Geranium (Pelargonium graveolens)

Practical Uses: see Geranium (Pelargonium graveolens)

Vibrational Influence: see Geranium (Pelargonium graveolens)

Emotional Influence: see Geranium (Pelargonium graveolens)

Synergistic to: see Geranium (Pelargonium graveolens)

Chakra Correspondence: see Geranium (Pelargonium graveolens)

Cosmetic Use: see Geranium (Pelargonium graveolens)

Source and Parts Used: leaves of the aromatic flowering plant

Ginger (Zingiber officinale)

Scent: pungent, spicy, warm

Clinical Uses: inflammatory conditions / debility and low body temperature / sluggish circulation / systemic candida / weak peristalsis of the digestive tract / arthritis / back pain and general musculoskeletal pain / weak appetite / sluggish lymph / blood clot prevention / blood vessel inflammation / high blood pressure / alcohol and substance cravings / mild-moderate depression / fatigue due to everyday stress / colds and influenza / weak immunity with over-stressed adrenal glands / low energy due to depression and everyday stress / Raynaud's Syndrome / chilblains / sexual debility / motion sickness and general nausea / nausea from chemotherapy / male impotence and low female sex drive / intestinal spasms and diarrhea / coughs

Body Systems Affected: musculoskeletal, immune, digestive, nervous/limbic, endocrine, circulatory, lymphatic, respiratory

Inhalation Effect: lifts depression / provides energy during afternoon slumps / potential to reduce cravings for alcohol and other addictive substances / releases the neurotransmitter dopamine in the brain and reduces symptoms of depression in some individuals / stimulates appetite

Dermal Effect: lowers blood pressure / decreases inflammation of blood vessels/ may be helpful in preventing blood clots / relieves pain in muscles, joints, ligaments, and tendons due to injury, overuse, and chronic pain syndromes such as fibromyalgia / helps reduce inflammation and pain due to arthritis and rheumatic conditions / stimulates stagnant lymph / warms the body by stimulating circulation / excellent oil to use during winter months to prevent chilblains / useful for Raynaud's Syndrome / increases peristalsis of the digestive system and helpful for constipation / stimulates the immune system / brings blood-flow to sexual organs and increases libido and pleasure / helps clear up diarrhea, flatulence, bloating, and intestinal spasms and pain when diluted and applied on the lower abdomen

/ balances intestinal flora especially after antibiotic use and also excellent for systemic candida / restores the body during or after everyday stress and depletion / helps break up respiratory congestion when added to chest rub formulas, especially when combined with pine needle essential oil / can be diluted and applied to the abdomen consistently every hour or two to decrease stubborn nausea from chemotherapy

Practical Uses: a few drops applied neat to the soles of the feet will warm the body during cold, winter months / makes a wonderful household cleaner (see Household Uses)

Vibrational Influence: inspires ambition and enthusiasm

Emotional Influence: reduces mental and emotional exhaustion

Synergistic to: clove, cardamom, peppermint, juniper berry, lemongrass

Chakra Correspondence: root, naval/sacral, solar plexus

Cosmetic Use: stimulates circulation, therefore useful for reducing the appearance of cellulite

Source and Parts Used: rhizomes of the plant

Caution: *Do not use during a fever or by anyone taking certain medications including blood thinners. Because ginger lowers blood pressure, people on medication should use ginger with caution as it may affect the prescribed required dosage. Those who are cautioned to avoid the intake of ginger in the diet due to medication contraindications should also avoid dermal use of ginger oil. Hemophiliacs should not use ginger essential oil. Ginger, both as a supplement and essential oil, may decrease available serotonin which can interfere with pharmaceutical antidepressants. Individuals with moderate-severe adrenal exhaustion should use ginger sparingly as not to overwork already-exhausted adrenal reserves. Avoid direct sunlight and tanning beds on exposed skin for up to 48 hours after using ginger oil dermally.*

Tip: Ginger essential oil, like myrrh and lavender, will enhance the properties of any essential oils mixed with it.

Goldenrod (Solidago canadensis)

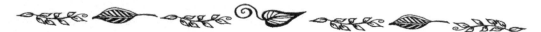

Scent: pungent and pleasantly herbaceous

Clinical Uses: liver support / allergies and seasonal allergies / respiratory infections / urinary tract infections / high blood pressure / nervous system balance / diabetes / tachycardia / male impotence

Body Systems Affected: endocrine, immune, respiratory, urinary, circulatory/cardiovascular, nervous

Inhalation Effect: calms and balances the nervous system

Dermal Effect: provides liver support especially in cases of congested liver / supports the immune system, especially helpful in combatting lung infections / helps lessen seasonal allergies and allergies to pet dander and environmental triggers / improves circulation and shown to be helpful for male impotence and premature ejaculation / an ally for urinary tract infections / helps the pancreas secrete insulin and useful for diabetic conditions / **Tip:** Apply 1-2 drops neat to the soles of the feet for all of the above

Practical Uses: N/A

Vibrational Influence: encourages the fortitude to live and speak one's truth / promotes resilience and survival / helps one to accept his or her sexuality / carries the energy of agape or universal brotherhood / supports the heart and high heart chakras

Emotional Influence: minimizes the need for approval of others and promotes selfhood / helps one to yield and allow

Synergistic to: carrot seed, yarrow

Chakra Correspondence: root, solar plexus, heart, throat

Cosmetic Use: beneficial for acne

Source and Parts Used: flowers and leaves of the meadow plant

Caution: *Diabetics should use goldenrod with caution, for it can alter the required dose of insulin or medication when used dermally; individuals with non-diabetic/reactive hypoglycemia should avoid dermal use of goldenrod essential oil*

Notes: The goldenrod plant is a major problem during allergy season for

many individuals with seasonal allergies/hay fever, but despite this, goldenrod essential oil has shown *significant ability* to *decrease* symptoms.

Grapefruit, Organic (Citrus paradisi)

Scent: fresh grapefruit, bright citrus

Clinical Uses: edema / weight loss / food cravings / sluggish or overburdened liver / weak appetite / mild-moderate depression / sluggish lymphatic system / tumors / Alzheimer's disease / acne / systemic candida-yeast overgrowth / PMS bloating and cravings / alcohol and drug recovery

Body Systems Affected: nervous/limbic, dermal, urinary, endocrine, lymphatic, circulatory

Inhalation Effect: eases symptoms of mild-moderate depression / improves outlook on rainy days and Mondays / reduces sugar and other food cravings / sharpens memory and improves brain function, especially in cases of Alzheimer's disease and other forms of dementia by inhibiting cholinesterase, the enzyme responsible for breaking down the neurotransmitter acetylcholine / sharpens focus and mental performance before exams, public speaking, or performances / increases neurotransmitters in the brain responsible for a sense of wellbeing / reduces cravings for alcohol and other substances

Dermal Effect: stimulates liver, gallbladder, kidneys, and lymph and helps to remove toxins / increases metabolism of fats / useful for weight loss and appearance of cellulite / promotes clearer skin due to its ability to remove toxins from the body / may have potential to shrink certain malignant and non-malignant tumors due to its high content of limonene / decreases candida in the body / balances oily skin / disinfects and helpful for acne / reduces water retention

Practical Uses: makes a wonderful and effective household cleaner

Vibrational Influence: lifts mental and emotional heaviness / encourages diligence

Emotional Influence: brightens outlook / encourages optimism

Synergistic to: bergamot, lemongrass

Chakra Correspondence: navel/sacral, brow

Cosmetic Use: ingredients in soaps, lotions, and other cosmetics designed for oily skin and hair

Source and Parts Used: cold-pressed fruit peels

Caution: Individuals on medications for viral infections, high cholesterol, high blood pressure, or heart conditions should avoid using dermal applications of grapefruit essential oil. If your doctor or pharmacist has recommended that you do not ingest grapefruit or other citrus while you are on specific medications, avoiding grapefruit essential oil is advisable. Avoid direct sunlight for 24 hours after dermal use.

Tip: *To avoid irritation, it is recommended to double or triple dilute when applied to skin other than the soles of the feet. To avoid pesticides in this cold-pressed essential oil, purchase organic grapefruit essential oil for dermal application.*

Helichrysum (Helichrysum italicum)

a.k.a as Immortelle & Everlasting

Scent: pungent and herbaceous with minty and fruity undertones

Clinical Uses: nerve regeneration / natural chelation of heavy metals / inflammatory conditions / injuries, wounds and burns / TMJ syndrome / skin repair / fatigue and debility after viral illness / herpes virus / blood clots / atherosclerosis and arteriosclerosis / psoriasis / scar tissue / physical-emotional-psychological trauma / headaches / IBS (irritable bowel syndrome) / asthma and bronchitis / rheumatoid arthritis / deep vein thrombosis

Body Systems Affected: nervous, urinary, musculoskeletal, integumentary, circulatory, digestive, respiratory

Inhalation Effect: eases symptoms of depression and anxiety related to trauma / reduces general anxiety

Dermal Effect: diluted and rubbed on the temples and forehead for headaches / diluted and rubbed on abdomen for IBS / diluted and rubbed onto the chest for asthma and coughs / removes heavy metals from the body and reduces the risk for atherosclerosis and arteriosclerosis (use neat on the soles of the feet) / reduces scar tissue / soothes psoriasis and is excellent for skin repair / potential to regenerate nerves/ eases TMJ pain and swelling when applied externally to jaw and neck / may prevent or hasten recovery from viral infection including herpes strains / helps deep vein thrombosis

Practical Uses: excellent First-Aid oil and can be applied undiluted to burns, cuts, sprains, strains, wounds, and boils

Vibrational Influence: heals the wounds of the soul by changing subconscious patterns

Emotional Influence: helps to confront and resolve deep psychological trauma / reduces anxiety / may be useful for PTSD (post-traumatic stress disorder)

Synergistic to: German chamomile, lavender

Chakra Correspondence: root, navel/sacral, heart, crown

Cosmetic Use: reduces the appearance of wrinkles

Source and Parts Used: flowering tops of the plant

Hyssop (Hyssop officinalis)

Scent: herbaceous and slightly sweet

Clinical Uses: emphysema / symptoms of multiple sclerosis / respiratory infections / lung, pancreas and spleen support / edema / melancholy depression / nervousness and states of hysteria or panic / herpes simplex and other viral infections / chronic nervous conditions / unstable blood pressure / sluggish digestion / poor mental concentration / food sensitivities or allergies that affect the digestive and respiratory systems

Body Systems Affected: respiratory, endocrine, nervous/limbic, immune, urinary, gastrointestinal

Inhalation Effect: sharpens brain power and memory / calms and balances nervous extremes / lifts outlook and mood / combats viruses when diffused via nebulizer / when diffused, maybe useful for allergies that affect the sinuses and lungs

Dermal Effect: combats viral infections / acts as a gentle diuretic and reduces edema / nourishes and increases energy of the pancreas, lungs, and spleen / helpful for high or low blood pressure or blood pressure that swings high and low / improves appetite, reduces bloating, and helps indigestion / soothes nervous stomach and digestive issues related to emotions or nervousness / effective when diluted and applied to chest and throat for sensitivities and allergies / effective when diluted and applied to abdomen for sensitivities and allergies to certain foods

Practical Uses: may be useful as a study aid

Vibrational Influence: provides protection / enforces energetic boundaries

Emotional Influence: lifts a broken, tired spirit / reduces melancholy

Synergistic to: sweet marjoram, geranium, lavender

Chakra Correspondence: navel/sacral, solar plexus, heart, brow

Cosmetic Use: N/A

Source and Parts Used: leaves and flowering tops of the aromatic plant

Caution: *Epileptics and anyone prone to seizures of any kind should not use hyssop essential oil. Do not use while pregnant or nursing.*

Tip: *Dilute well, especially with sensitive skin.*

Jasmine Absolute (Jasminum officinale, J. sambac, J. grandiflorum)

Scent: sweet, hypnotic floral with vanilla undertones

Clinical Uses: female hormone imbalance / PMS / painful menstruation / anxiety / symptoms of mild-moderate depression and apathy / impaired liver function / nervous exhaustion / Chronic Fatigue Syndrome / childbirth and post-partum depression / male impotence / weak orgasmic response in women

Body Systems Affected: endocrine, nervous

Inhalation Effect: calms the nerves / decreases female sexual inhibition, increases libido and orgasmic capacity in women / lifts the spirits / helps women in labor to experience less pain and shorter delivery time / very useful to prevent and ease symptoms of post-partum depression / supports men's erectile function

Dermal Effect: may be useful for hepatitis and impaired function of the liver / regulates female hormones and useful for PMS and menstrual pain

Practical Uses: may help to prevent and treat head lice

Vibrational Influence: attracts higher frequencies and energies / cultivates harmony

Emotional Influence: helps resolve trauma from emotional abuse / calms agitation and fears / inspires confidence in one's physical self and sexuality / heightens the senses / lessens misplaced guilt / improves self-worth / inspires creativity

Synergistic to: ylang ylang, geranium, clary sage

Chakra Correspondence: root, navel/sacral, solar plexus, heart, brow

Cosmetic Use: used in lotions, cleansers, conditioners, and shampoos to balance combination, irritated, and oily skin / for dry skin and hair / according to some sources, strengthens hair and stimulates hair growth when applied to the roots.

Source and Parts Used: flowers from the shrub

Tip: Jasmine flower is one of the most adulterated as well as chemically simulated oils. Be sure to purchase from a reputable supplier and never settle for inexpensive fakes. Use sparingly, for one drop goes a long way and can be overpowering if used in larger quantities. This rather expensive oil can be purchased in affordable diluted form and possesses the same properties and beautiful scent.

Juniper Berry (Juniperus communis)

Scent: pungent, bright evergreen with fruity undertones

Clinical Uses: sciatica / neuropathy/ nerve damage / cystitis / chronic stress / arthritis / muscle and joint pain / diabetes / edema / persistent coughs / sluggish liver function / cirrhosis / infections especially those of the respiratory tract / sluggish lymph / skin rashes such as weeping eczema due to toxins in the bloodstream / Parkinson's disease / addiction recovery

Body Systems Affected: nervous, immune, urinary, endocrine, respiratory, musculoskeletal, circulatory

Inhalation Effect: helps to relieve sinus infection, pain, and congestion / provides a nice "wake up" boost of energy on sluggish mornings or during afternoon slumps / opens up bronchial airways and provides a wonderful, cleansing steam in saunas when sprinkled on a wet washcloth or towel / renews body and spirit after a long work day or period of stress / excellent to reduce or eliminate sinus pain from allergies or cold weather, especially when used as a steam with white thyme essential oil / may be helpful in nourishing the adrenals and supply of neurotransmitters, therefore reducing cravings associated with substance addiction

Dermal Effect: reduces water retention / helps nerves to regenerate / improves communication between nerves / fights colds, flu, sinus infections, and bronchitis when diluted and rubbed on the chest / supports and stimulates better liver and kidney function/ excellent oil for bladder infections / cleanses the blood and may be useful for certain types of eczema stemming from built-up toxins, food sensitivies, and excessive chemicals in the diet / valuable remedy for muscle and joint pain and that associated with chronic pain syndromes / stimulates circulation of both blood and lymph / may be highly useful and effective for cases of neuropathy / lowers blood sugar and useful for diabetics / for nervous depletion and periods of stress / may be helpful for Parkinson's disease

Practical Uses: effective and fragrant disinfectant when used in a nebulizer to cleanse the air in sick rooms / a few drops added to a wet washcloth or towel in a sauna will create a cleansing steam / also excellent oil to add to baths, footbaths, and showers / makes a wonderful ingredient in household cleaners, natural potpourris, and room sprays / a drop or two added to final rinse water when washing hair will help control dandruff

Vibrational Influence: cleansing and protective / cleanses the energy field and environment of malevolent energies

Emotional Influence: instills a sense of stability / inspires optimism

Synergistic to: pine bark, pine needle, basil

Chakra Correspondence: root, solar plexus, heart, brow

Cosmetic Use: added to shampoos to control dandruff

Source and Parts Used: berries of the evergreen shrub

Caution: *Juniper berry, though helpful for strengthening the kidneys, should be avoided by those with kidney disease. Individuals with severe reactive/non-diabetic hypoglycemia (low blood sugar) should use juniper sparingly in dermal applications. Diabetics should also use this oil with caution, for it may affect required dosage of insulin.*

Lavender (Lavandula angustifolia)

a.k.a. as true lavender

Scent: herbaceous and floral without overpowering sweetness

Clinical Uses: boosting immunity / First-Aid / sunburn / seasonal and environmental allergies / asthma / prevention of bruising and swelling / injuries, sprains, and strains / nervous system conditions / healing of wounds, cuts, scrapes, burns, pimples, boils, and insect bites / soft-tissue injuries / homeostasis of the body / insomnia / anxiety and panic / blood sugar balance / high blood pressure or erratic blood pressure / viral and bacterial infections, cold, and flu / certain skin cancers / food cravings / serotonin deficiency / prevention and treatment of burns before or after radiation treatment / diaper rash

Body Systems Affected: immune, dermal, endocrine, nervous/limbic

Inhalation Effect: calms the body and curbs severe anxiety / reduces insomnia, poor sleep, and racing thoughts / gently brings the body out of physical shock / stimulates serotonin and helps the body to utilize this neurotransmitter / minimizes sugar and starch cravings / natural antihistamine, especially effective when combined with Roman chamomile, provided the person is not allergic to chamomile or plants in the ragweed family / helps to calm trembling and shakiness / kills bacteria and viruses when diffused into the air via nebulizer

Dermal Effect: brings equilibrium to the body and calms extremes / highly effective for infections, cold, and flu / builds resistance and reduces allergies and sensitivities / soothes and heals sunburn / heals wounds, cuts, burns, and scrapes / the primary oil to use for First-Aid and be used neat / apply to temples, forehead and back of the neck for tension or nervous headaches / may prevent and reduce certain skin cancers, especially when combined with frankincense essential oil / will kill yeast and fungal infections of the skin or feet when used in footbaths / beneficial for balancing high or erratic blood pressure when applied neat to the soles of the feet / will help to balance blood sugar if it is on the low side and useful for individuals with reactive/non-diabetic hypoglycemia when applied neat to the soles of the feet or the palms of the hands / will calm trembling and inner shaking when applied neat to the soles of the feet or the palms of the hands / can prevent or minimize burns from radiation treatments if applied beforehand, especially combined with Roman and German chamomile essential oils / may be diluted and applied singularly or combined with Roman chamomile to soothe baby's diaper rash

Practical Uses: First-Aid (see pages 55 & 66) / a drop or two in water for household plants to fight molds and fungus / room spray / effective household cleaner / treats and kills head lice / guards against fleas / insect repellant including mosquitoes and flies / nice scent to use for clothes when sprinkled generously onto a damp wash cloth and added with wet clothes in the dryer

Vibrational Influence: restores people and energies to a state of equilibrium / clears the energy field

Emotional Influence: calms adrenalin and the fight or flight response / instantly calms the limbic portion of the brain, namely the amygdala, thus lessening panic and fear in the psyche and the body / effective for cases of emotional shock, especially when combined with neroli or ylang ylang / helps us to process and integrate the past and emotional wounds of childhood / eases feelings of resentment

Synergistic to: helichrysum, frankincense, neroli, ylang ylang

Chakra Correspondence: root, solar plexus, heart, crown

Cosmetic Use: numerous uses in cosmetics, soaps, cleansers, skin balms, and perfumes / balances combination skin

Source and Parts Used: flowering tops of the fragrant plant

Caution: *Individuals with severe low blood pressure should not overuse lavender. Though rare, allergy to lavender can occur in certain individuals and can cause itchy skin rashes. In this case, triple dilute or only apply neat (undiluted) to the soles of the feet.*

Tip: Clinically, lavender essential oil is perhaps the most valuable and versatile of all essential oils. Lavender essential oil is wonderful for First-Aid, and a few drops can be applied directly into a cut to minimize and stop bleeding, as well as disinfect the area. For individuals with reactive/non-diabetic hypoglycemia (low blood sugar), a drop or two on the palms of the hands and applied along the spine will stop shakiness and other unpleasant symptoms; this is effective for times when the blood sugar falls due to skipped meals, too much sugar and carbohydrates, too little protein, too little sleep, or emotional stress. This method is enhanced when combined with a drop of frankincense.

Lavender, Spike (Lavandula latifolia)

Scent: sharper and more camphorous than Lavandula angustifolia (true lavender)

Clinical Uses: rheumatic pain / disinfecting wounds / digestive distress / infections

Body Systems Affected: immune, dermal, respiratory, gastrointestinal, nervous

Inhalation Effect: calms nerves and brightens the mood / combats respiratory infections

Dermal Effect: powerful disinfectant of cuts and wounds / calms intestinal distress and bloating

Practical Uses: repels insects

Vibrational Influence: cleanses lower energies and frequencies / carries healing and nurturing energy of the earth and the Sacred Feminine

Emotional Influence: instills calm without dulling sense of alertness / inspires compassion and reconciliation / lessens worry / minimizes potentially toxic emotions such as jealousy and bitterness

Synergistic to: geranium, lemon

Chakra Correspondence: root, navel/sacral

Cosmetic Use: acts as an astringent for the skin when diluted and added to water in a spray bottle

Source and Parts Used: flowering tops of the fragrant plant

Note: It is believed that spike lavender is a natural cross between true lavender and sage

<u>Ledum</u> a.k.a. Greenland Moss (Ledum groenlandicum)

Scent: pungent and herbaceous

Clinical Uses: liver support and protection / Lyme disease / thyroid balance for both hypothyroid and hyperthyroid conditions / nausea from chemotherapy treatments

Body Systems Affected: endocrine, immune, nervous

Inhalation Effect: calms the nerves

Dermal Effect: helps to lessen nausea and vomiting after chemotherapy treatments / helps the liver to filter toxins and renew itself after illness or addiction / supports the balance of thyroid hormones / boosts the immune system / helps the liver and kidneys to filter more efficiently after chemotherapy / may be very beneficial in combatting Lyme disease and other tick-borne illnesses

Practical Uses: N/A

Vibrational Influence: cleanses energy fields of people and place of toxins

Emotional Influence: helps one to acknowledge and honor deeply-held or buried emotions

Synergistic to: cardamom, German chamomile

Chakra Correspondence: root, solar plexus, throat

Cosmetic Use: N/A

Source and Parts Used: leaves and flowers from the rhododendron shrub also known as Labrador Tea.

Lemon, Organic (Citrus limonum)

Scent: fresh citrus, bright and clean

Clinical Uses: stimulation of white blood cells / viral and bacterial infections / pneumonia / anemia / deep vein thrombosis / warts / staph infection / tumors / breast cysts and breast cancer / arteriosclerosis / high blood pressure / parasites / sluggish circulation / varicose veins / mild-moderate depression / obesity / sluggish lymph / overburdened or fatty liver / edema / cleanses the kidneys and blood / systemic candida / poor eyesight due to tension and stress

Body Systems Affected: immune, circulatory, nervous, lymphatic, urinary

Inhalation Effect: elevates mood and promotes psychological wellbeing

Dermal Effect: stimulates white blood cell production and boosts immunity against serious infections such as staph / kills viruses and bacteria when diffused into the air via nebulizer / clears up warts by killing the virus that causes them / helps to flush the liver of toxins and cleanses the kidneys / reduces fluid retention / normalizes high blood pressure, especially when combined with lavender / helps to normalize and restore intestinal flora, reducing harmful yeast / applied neat to the soles of the feet, may greatly improve eyesight / supports breast health when diluted and rubbed onto the breasts, especially when combined with frankincense applied up to 5x a week

Practical Uses: household cleaner, par excellence / a few drops added to a glass of unclean water will combat viruses and bacteria on contact / tick repellant

Vibrational Influence: brings light where there is darkness, hope where there is despair / holds the energy of new beginnings

Emotional Influence: eases feelings of hopelessness / lifts depression

Synergistic to: lavender, geranium, clove, tea tree

Chakra Correspondence: root, solar plexus, heart

Cosmetic Use: used in cosmetics, soaps, and shampoos to balance oily skin and hair

Source and Parts Used: cold-pressed fruit peels

Caution: *Lemon essential oil can cause skin sensitivity when applied prior to sun or tanning bed exposure. Please wait 48 hours before exposing skin to either direct sunlight or tanning beds. Lemon can also cause skin rashes in dermal blends and/or baths. Please dilute well. Individuals on blood thinners should avoid dermal use of lemon essential oil.*

Tip: It is recommended to use organic lemon essential oil, especially for dermal use to avoid absorbing pesticides from the cold-pressed peels. Organic lemon essential oil should be in every traveler's carry-on bag or suitcase. A few drops added to a glass of unclean water will kill viruses and bacteria and make the water safer—if not safe—to drink.

Notes: Reputable studies since 1970 show that compounds in lemon essential oil are thousands of times stronger than chemotherapy and do not adversely affect healthy cells. These compounds have also been proven to slow the growth of cancer cells in twelve cancers including breast, prostate, colon, lung, and pancreas. Lemon essential oil diluted and combined with frankincense essential oil makes a nourishing and supportive blend to rub on the breasts to keep cysts and disease at bay. When combined with ginger, lemon essential oil makes an excellent combination to help remove toxins from the body and can be applied neat to the soles of the feet- (It is recommended to drink plenty of water for a few hours after this application in order for toxins to be flushed from the system.)

<u>Lemongrass</u> (Cymbopogon citrates)

Scent: bright, grassy citrus with citronella undertones

Clinical Uses: anemia / athlete's foot and other fungal infections / systemic candida / viral infections / edema / pain and inflammation / adrenal weakness and debility / vascular weakness / weak connective tissue / weak

or torn ligaments / poor lymphatic flow / sluggish circulation / depression and despondency / infectious fevers / overstimulated nervous system / MRSA / Lupus

Body Systems Affected: immune, circulatory, endocrine, musculoskeletal,

Inhalation Effect: brightens the spirits and instills ambition / combats viruses, bacteria, and molds when diffused into the air via nebulizer / calms the nervous system

Dermal Effect: helps to strengthen vascular walls / builds the blood / reduces water retention / decreases pain / decreases systemic inflammation / fights viruses and bacteria / strengthens connective tissue throughout the body / supports and nourishes the adrenals / improves circulation / calms and balances the nervous system / will support the body in cases of Lupus / helpful for compromised ligaments when applied diluted

Practical Uses: makes an effective mosquito and tick repellant, especially when combined with geranium essential oil / excellent household cleaner / 1 drop added to a cup of warm water makes a pleasant and effective mouthwash / disinfects the air when diffused via nebulizer / nice scent to use for clothes when sprinkled generously onto a damp wash cloth and added with wet clothes in the dryer / flea repellant

Vibrational Influence: raises frequency and clears the energy field

Emotional Influence: stimulates feelings of happiness and hope

Synergistic to: geranium, eucalyptus radiata, basil, rosewood

Chakra Correspondence: root, solar plexus

Cosmetic Use: added to soaps for antimicrobial action / minute amounts used in perfumery

Source and Parts Used: leaves of the fragrant grass

Caution: Dermal use of *lemongrass essential oil should be avoided by those on certain medications including blood thinners. May cause photosensitivity; avoid direct sunlight and tanning beds on exposed skin for 24 hours after dermal application.*

Lemon Verbena (Lippia citriodora)

Scent: bright lemon with fruity and woody undertones

Clinical Uses: nervous exhaustion / symptoms of depression / digestive upsets related to nerves or emotions / Crohn's disease

Body Systems Affected: nervous/limbic, gastrointestinal

Inhalation Effect: improves mental function and makes an excellent study aid / improves the production and utilization of specific neurotransmitters needed to elevate mood and outlook / calms a nervous belly

Dermal Effect: tonic for the nervous system and increases cellular life force of the nerves / calms an agitated, nervous stomach when diluted and applied to abdomen / may be helpful for Crohn's disease when diluted and applied to abdomen up to 3x a week or daily for a period of time

Practical Uses: effective study aid

Vibrational Influence: brings harmony and equilibrium to people and spaces

Emotional Influence: combats depression of all types / promotes joy / alleviates exaggerated, misplaced guilt

Synergistic to: melissa (lemon), lemongrass

Chakra Correspondence: solar plexus, brow

Cosmetic Use: a delightful fragrance often added to soaps, cleansers, and perfumes

Source and Parts Used: leaves of the fragrant plant

Caution: *Avoid direct sunlight and tanning beds for up to 72 hours after dermal application.*

Lime (Citrus aurantifolia)

Scent: citrus with green undertones

Clinical Uses: exhausted nervous system / stomach pain and digestive sluggishness / lung congestion / sluggish or overburdened liver / weak appetite / poor circulation of blood and lymph

Body Systems Affected: immune, circulatory, nervous, lymphatic, urinary

Inhalation Effect: opens breathing passages when used in a hot steam / lifts the spirits / tonic for the nervous system / stimulates a healthy appetite / sore throat

Dermal Effect: helps promote circulation of both blood and lymph when small amounts are used in massage or applied neat to the soles of the feet / boosts immunity / helps the liver clear out toxins from a diet of processed foods, excessive alcohol or high sugar consumption / calms a griping belly when diluted and applied to abdomen / fights sore throat when diluted and applied dermally to neck and throat area

Practical Uses: excellent household cleaner

Vibrational Influence: cleanses built-up emotions and energies from spaces after arguments

Emotional Influence: lifts depression and apathy

Synergistic to: lemon, mandarin, orange, tangerine, lemongrass, melissa (lemon balm)

Chakra Correspondence: solar plexus, heart, throat

Cosmetic Use: used in soaps and perfumery

Source and Parts Used: cold-pressed fruit peels

Caution: *Avoid direct sunlight and tanning beds for up to 48 hours after dermal application. Individuals on blood thinners should avoid dermal use of lime essential oil.*

Tip: Look *for steam distilled* (versus cold-pressed) lime essential oil to avoid or lessen photosensitivity. Organic lime essential oil is best for dermal use.

Mandarin (Citrus reticulata)

Scent: sweet tangerine-like citrus

Clinical Uses: children's restlessness, anxiety, and stress / ADHD in children and adults / metabolism of fats / sluggish digestion in children and adults / overburdened liver

Body Systems Affected: nervous, dermal, gastrointestinal, endocrine

Inhalation Effect: calms a racing mind and tense body in both children and adults / improves mood / soothes anxiety especially when combined with neroli or ylang ylang

Dermal Effect: nourishing and calming to the digestive system when diluted and applied to abdomen / improves metabolism of fats when applied neat to the soles of the feet / prevents stretch marks / gently helps the liver to filter toxins

Practical Uses: household cleaners and fragrant room sprays or air fresheners

Vibrational Influence: ushers in harmony on multidimensional levels

Emotional Influence: carries the energy of hope and peace / calms and restores emotionally-exhausted minds and hearts / gently brings us to the present moment when we tend toward living in the past

Synergistic to: tangerine, orange, rose

Chakra Correspondence: solar plexus, heart

Cosmetic Use: minimizes and helps prevent stretch marks during pregnancy when diluted and rubbed onto the belly and other areas; for best results, dilute and combine with lavender in a nourishing carrier oil such as jojoba, evening primrose, or sesame / used in soaps, cleansers, and toners for oily skin / excellent to add to cleansers for teenage acne

Source and Parts Used: cold-pressed fruit peels

Caution: *Mandarin essential oil can cause skin sensitivity if applied dermally prior to direct sun exposure or tanning beds. Please wait 24-48 hours before skin is exposed to sunlight or tanning beds. Individuals on blood thinners should avoid dermal use of mandarin essential oil.*

Tip: The oil is cold-pressed from fruit rinds therefore purchasing organic essential oil for dermal applications will prevent the absorption of pesticides

Notes: Mandarin is the same species as tangerine, and these two citrus oils are often assumed to be one and the same, but their essential oils offer different benefits. Mandarin essential oil tends to be greenish in color, while tangerine can be a bright orange. Mandarin, like tangerine, is a premiere essential oil for children. It is gentle, effective, and pleasing. It is also one of the few essential oils considered safe to use during pregnancy, provided the scent is pleasing to the mother-to-be. Mandarin is also a valuable and uplifting essential oil for seniors.

Marjoram, Sweet (Origanum majorana)

Scent: lesser quality: pungent with oregano-like undertones; high-quality: includes sourcing the flowering tops which yields a delightfully sweet, herbaceous oil with perfume-like undertones

Clinical Uses: stress-related exhaustion / menstrual pain / headaches / high blood pressure / nervous tension / physical symptoms associated with deep longing, grief, and sadness / muscles aches and strains / rheumatoid arthritis / fibromyalgia pain / coughs / phobias

Body Systems Affected: circulatory / nervous / musculoskeletal / nervous/limbic

Inhalation Effect: eases coughs and congestion of lungs and sinuses / induces calm / soothes grief-stricken heart and mind / prepares the body and mind for sleep / lifts symptoms of depression / comforts feelings of isolation and loneliness / helpful for diminishing phobias and preoccupation with them

Dermal Effect: eases coughs when diluted and rubbed onto the chest / warms muscles and good to use after exertion or workouts / decreases pain and brings circulation to muscle strains / lessens pain from rheumatoid arthritis, fibromyalgia, and chronic pain syndromes

Practical Uses: household cleaner

Vibrational Influence: holds the energy of comfort and gentle perseverance

Emotional Influence: for deep longing, grief, and sadness / lifts a spirit burdened by worry, melancholy, and despair / soothes depressive states / encourages a shift in perspective to feel contentment / helps to ease obsessive thoughts / comforting during times of loneliness

Synergistic to: lavender, spearmint, melissa (lemon balm)

Chakra Correspondence: solar plexus, heart, high heart

Cosmetic Use: N/A

Source and Parts Used: leaves and flowering tops

Caution: *Individuals on blood thinners should avoid dermal use of marjoram essential oil.*

Tip: Marjoram, translated from the Greek, means "joy of the mountains."

May Chang (Litsea cubeba)

a.k.a. Litsea

Scent: lemon-like with grassy undertones

Clinical Uses: excessive perspiration / flatulence and abdominal discomfort / insomnia or disrupted sleep / irregular heartbeat / high blood pressure / lung cancer

Body Systems Affected: dermal, gastrointestinal, nervous, circulatory

Inhalation Effect: reduces blood pressure when too high / lessens excessive perspiration / induces sleep especially when inhaled with lavender / calms the nerves and has potential to calm irregular heartbeat / could be an ally for lung cancer

Dermal Effect: balances blood pressure / calms flatulence and other digestive disturbances when diluted and applied to the abdomen / promotes sleep and relaxation, especially when blended with Roman chamomile and lavender

Practical Uses: household cleaner with clean, lemon-like freshness

Vibrational Influence: cleans away energetic debris from conflicts

Emotional Influence: balances emotional extremes / calms the mind and intrusive thoughts

Synergistic to: Roman chamomile, lemon, tangerine

Chakra Correspondence: navel/sacral, solar plexus, heart

Cosmetic Use: fragrance for soaps and perfumes

Source and Parts Used: seeds of the tropical tree

Notes: May chang essential oil has been shown to combat lung cancer cells. The essential oil can be a substitution for more pungent lemongrass essential oil.

Melissa (Melissa officinalis)

a.k.a. Lemon Balm

Scent: lemon-like with grassy overtones

Clinical Uses: hyperthyroidism / herpes simplex / weak immunity / nervous disorders / nervous depression / high blood pressure / shock / irregular menstruation

Body Systems Affected: immune, nervous/limbic, circulatory

Inhalation Effect: promotes profound, deep relaxation / lowers blood pressure / helps to bring the body out of shock / may minimize allergy symptoms / eases symptoms of mild-moderate depression and melancholy

Dermal Effect: helps to clear and prevent herpes simplex outbreaks / helpful for cold sores when diluted a bit and applied directly to blisters / lowers blood pressure / helps decrease and balance excessive thyroid hormone / balancing to the menstrual cycle when regularly applied neat to the soles of the feet

Practical Uses: may be helpful for allergies

Vibrational Influence: holds energy of youthful enthusiasm and renewal

Emotional Influence: helps the heart and psyche to recover sense of self and heal from emotional abuse / encourages hopeful outlook / comforts a

grief-stricken spirit / especially comforting and helpful for women during hormonal shifts and transitions / eases symptoms of deep melancholy

Synergistic to: geranium, lavender, sweet marjoram

Chakra Correspondence: root, heart, throat

Cosmetic Use: used in toiletries and perfumes

Source and Parts Used: leaves and stems of the aromatic plant

Caution: *Individuals on blood thinners should avoid dermal use of melissa/lemon balm essential oil. Individuals with hypothyroidism (low thyroid) should not use melissa essential oil long-term.*

Tips: Beware of imitation melissa essential oil; many products labeled as melissa or lemon balm are made from or diluted with citronella and lemongrass essential oils and do not offer melissa's unique and powerful properties or scent. This rather expensive oil can be purchased in affordable diluted form and possesses the same properties and aroma.

Myrrh (Commiphora myrrha)

Scent: woody and resinous with subtle smoky undertones

Clinical Uses: hypothyroidism / kidney support during and after chemotherapy / prevention of UV ray damage and possibly skin cancer such as melanoma / fungal and bacterial infections / systemic candida / high cholesterol / wound care / gingivitis / nervousness, trembling, or upset stomach from intense emotions / menstrual imbalances

Body Systems Affected: nervous, immune, integumentary, reproductive

Inhalation Effect: increases oxygen to the brain / is known to be helpful for hypothyroidism when inhaled daily for 5-10 minutes first thing in the morning / calms the body and mind after confrontation or other emotional upsets / directly influences and balances the hypothalamus in the brain / calms the amygdala, the part of the brain that governs emotions, fear, and decision-making and plays a vital role in the physiological responses that trigger anxiety and panic attacks

Dermal Effect: helps the kidneys eliminate toxins during and after chemotherapy / beneficial and supportive of the skin; a small amount (1 drop) can be added to unscented lotions, aloe vera, or nourishing carrier oil such as jojoba or sesame / helps wounds heal quicker and better / combats systemic candida when applied to the soles of the feet / potential to lower high cholesterol / excellent for fungal infections / may regulate the menstrual period

Practical Uses: 1 drop or two added to warm water makes an excellent and healing mouthwash for sore gums, gingivitis, periodontitis, or a sore mouth after dental work / 1 drop of full-strength essential oil can also be added to toothpaste to fight plaque, freshen breath, and cleanse the mouth

Vibrational Influence: holds the energy of resilience, steadfastness, and survival even during the most adverse circumstances / provides fortitude and comfort during grief, the dying process, or life transitions that involve the death of old dreams, selves, and ways of living

Emotional Influence: helps one to transition through grief or death / calms the nerves / calms the body and mind when inhaled after hearing bad news or experiencing intense emotions / comforting and considered an ancient sacred substance which makes it the primary essential oil to use to help a person transition through death therefore extremely valuable for hospice work

Synergistic to: frankincense, Atlas cedarwood, sandalwood

Chakra Correspondence: base, solar plexus, heart, crown

Cosmetic Use: used in mouth washes / as a base note-fixative in perfumery

Source and Parts Used: resin from the tree

Tip: This rather expensive oil can be purchased in affordable diluted form and possesses the same properties and scent. Myrrh essential oil, like ginger, will enhance the properties of any essential oil mixed with it.

Myrtle, Green (Myrtus communis)

Scent: green and herbaceous with subtle eucalyptus-like undertones

Clinical Uses: hypothyroidism (low thyroid) / ovarian imbalances / asthma / lung support / children's coughs / psoriasis / prostate support

Body Systems Affected: endocrine, reproductive, respiratory

Inhalation Effect: beneficial for the lungs and improves breathing / mildly calming to the nerves and uplifting to the mood

Dermal Effect: may be helpful to balance low thyroid conditions when diluted and applied to the thyroid area and applied neat to the soles of the feet daily / decreases congestion and useful for children's coughs when diluted and rubbed onto the chest / supports the balance of female hormones when applied consistently to the soles of the feet (up to 3x a week) / supports the prostate when diluted and rubbed onto the lower back, sacrum, and abdomen

Practical Uses: fragrant addition to household cleaners and air fresheners

Vibrational Influence: brings clarity / sweeps out the old to usher in new beginnings / cleanses the energy field of people and places / holds the energetic vitality and healing force of the natural world

Emotional Influence: provides a quick "pick-me-up" and second wind in cases of emotional exhaustion

Synergistic to: clary sage, spearmint

Chakra Correspondence: root, navel/sacral, heart

Cosmetic Use: effective astringent for oily and acne-prone skin

Source and Parts Used: leaves of the bush

Neroli Absolute (Citrus aurantium, C. bigaradia, C. vulgaris)

Scent: sweet with "green" undertones

Clinical Uses: nervous conditions including insomnia, anxiety, panic attacks, and trembling / dementia / racing heart from nervousness or female hormonal shifts / skin rashes from an overstimulated or overburdened nervous system / symptoms of melancholy depression

Body Systems Affected: nervous, integumentary

Inhalation Effect: calms the fight or flight response and eases anxiety, panic attacks, obsessive worry, and dread / sharpens the mind and memory and may be helpful for certain types of dementia when inhaled daily / gently induces sleep in cases of insomnia / lifts depressive moods / highly effective for calming heart palpitations caused by female hormonal shifts / stops internal trembling and shaking almost immediately, especially when combined with ylang ylang essential oil / releases feel-good endorphins

Dermal Effect: calms an agitated body and spirit / reduces stretch marks and nourishing for skin rashes

Practical Uses: N/A

Vibrational Influence: invites higher frequencies-energies / makes room for joy and encourages our willingness to receive it

Emotional Influence: calms the nerves with almost immediate effect / minimizes physical symptoms caused by conscious or subconscious emotions / instills a sense of hope

Synergistic to: ylang ylang, lavender, frankincense

Chakra Correspondence: solar plexus, heart, brow, crown

Cosmetic Use: can be added to unscented lotion or carrier oil to reduce stretch marks / softens skin when diluted in lotion or carrier oil / used in perfumery

Source and Parts Used: blossoms of the orange tree, most often from the bitter orange also called Seville

Tip: This rather expensive oil can be purchased in affordable diluted form and possesses the same properties and scent. Do not confuse neroli with niaouli essential oil; the two are distinctly different.

Niaouli (Melaleuca quinquenervia viridiflora)

a.k.a. MQV and Gomenol

Scent: pungent and herbaceous with sweet menthol-like overtones

Clinical Uses: weak immunity / allergies / whooping cough and other respiratory conditions

Body Systems Affected: immune, respiratory

Inhalation Effect: may help to ease allergy symptoms / brightens the spirit when feeling blue from monotonous routine, Monday mornings, and rainy days

Dermal Effect: boosts immunity especially to fight viral infections / eases coughs, bronchitis, and laryngitis / effective as antibiotics when applied neat to the soles of the feet / may help ease allergy symptoms when applied neat to the soles of the feet or diluted and rubbed onto the chest and throat / has analgesic (pain-reducing) effects

Practical Uses: household cleaner

Vibrational Influence: protects the energy field of people and places from outside, unwanted energies and influences

Emotional Influence: uplifts the mood and encourages us to get things done on the to-do list

Synergistic to: eucalyptus, tea tree, ravensara

Chakra Correspondence: root, heart

Cosmetic Use: can be dabbed onto acne with a cotton swab

Source and Parts Used: leaves of the tree

Tip: Do not confuse niaouli with neroli essential oil; the two are distinctly different.

Nutmeg (Myristica fragrans)

Scent: pungent sweet spice with slightly medicinal undertones in its undiluted state

Clinical Uses: adrenal gland and nervous system support for times of stress / Cushing's syndrome / non-Addison's hypoadrenia / Crohn's disease / Alzheimer's disease / osteoarthritis / mental fatigue / tired or weak digestion / smoking cessation

Body Systems Affected: endocrine, nervous, gastrointestinal

Inhalation Effect: boosts physical energy if inhaled for short intervals / sharpens memory and improves mental function and concentration / may be helpful for symptoms of Alzheimer's disease / may be helpful for quitting smoking and reducing the cravings <u>Caution:</u> *do not inhale for long periods of time or habitually*

Dermal Effect: 1 drop diluted in carrier oil and applied to abdomen will improve digestion / 1 drop diluted in carrier oil and rubbed onto arthritis sites or sore muscles will ease pain and inflammation / stimulates the heart and the adrenals when used sparingly and diluted for massage / has a balancing effect on non-clinical (non-Addison's) hypoadrenia *and* Cushing's syndrome.

Practical Uses: lovely fragrance to add to potpourris and room sprays; 1 drop or 2 goes a long way

Vibrational Influence: encourages courage and self-confidence / promotes the will to survive / inspires self-reliance and practicality when life challenges us to the breaking point

Emotional Influence: encourages creative practicality, self-reliance, independence, and emotional strength / helps one dig down deeply to find strength during times of heartbreak

Synergistic to: ginger, juniper berry, balsam fir

Chakra Correspondence: root, navel/sacral, solar plexus

Cosmetic Use: used sparingly in perfumery

Source and Parts Used: egg-shaped seeds from the tree

Caution: *nutmeg essential oil, like the spice, is toxic in large doses; do not overuse dermally or inhale excessively. Do not add to bath water or footbaths. Nutmeg stimulates the heart and should be used sparingly or avoided by anyone with weak or compromised heart function.*

Tip: Brushing 1 drop of undiluted nutmeg and 1 drop of balsam fir or pine needle essential oil into the hair will linger most of the day and provide the body and mind with extra energy on heavily-scheduled work days.

Onycha See Benzoin

Orange, Sweet (Citrus sinensis)

Scent: like the fruit, sweet citrus

Clinical Uses: immune support / constipation / mild depression / sluggish circulation / some forms of anxiety including Obsessive Compulsive Disorder (OCD)

Body Systems Affected: immune, nervous/limbic, gastrointestinal, circulatory

Inhalation Effect: promotes cheerfulness and lifts symptoms of mild-moderate depression / can be diffused into the air via nebulizer to induce a sunny and calm atmosphere / may be helpful in killing bacteria, viruses, and mold spores when diffused into the air via nebulizer / may be helpful in cases of allergies / may be helpful for Obsessive Compulsive Disorder / minimizes obsessive and intrusive thoughts

Dermal Effect: enhances vitamin C absorption when applied to the soles of the feet / helps ease constipation when diluted and applied to the abdomen / potential to shrink malignant tumors / boosts the immune system when added neat to the soles of the feet, especially when applied with organic lemon or clove essential oil / improves circulation and may be helpful in preventing blood clots

Practical Uses: makes a wonderful household cleaner and room spray / can be added to natural potpourris for an invigorating and inviting scent

Vibrational Influence: sweeps away darkness of the past and gently invites us into the present moment with hopeful anticipation

Emotional Influence: encourages healthy self-assertion / minimizes symptoms of mild-moderate depression / takes the edge off frazzled nerves / encourages self-appreciation and self-forgiveness

Synergistic to: bergamot, Roman chamomile

Chakra Correspondence: root, navel/sacral, heart

Cosmetic Use: used in soaps, cleansers, shampoos and perfumery / balances oily skin when added to cleansers / gives tired, mature skin a pick-me-up

Source and Parts Used: cold-pressed from fruit peels

Caution: *Sweet orange essential oil can cause skin sensitivity if it is applied prior to direct sun exposure or tanning beds. Please wait 24-48 hours before skin is exposed to sunlight or tanning beds. Individuals on blood thinners should avoid dermal use of orange essential oil.*

Tip: Orange essential oil is cold-pressed from fruit rinds; purchase organic essential oil for dermal applications.

Oregano (Origanum vulgare)

Scent: pungent, herbaceous, and medicinal

Clinical Uses: Lyme disease / all viral, bacterial, and fungal infections / colds and flu / weak immunity / tonsillitis / combats E. coli, Salmonella and Pseudomonas bacteria / intestinal distress including infectious diarrhea, bloating, and discomfort / Epstein-Barr virus / parasites

Body Systems Affected: immune, gastrointestinal

Inhalation Effect: N/A (do not inhale)

Dermal Effect: apply 1 or 2 drops neat or diluted <u>only</u> to the soles of the feet for any bacterial, viral, or fungal infection, food poisoning, or intestinal distress; <u>*do not use for long periods of time*</u>

Practical Uses: makes a powerful addition to household spray cleaners

Vibrational Influence: combats malevolent energies

Emotional Influence: N/A

Synergistic to: clove, lemon, basil, sweet marjoram, white thyme, cinnamon bark

Chakra Correspondence: root, navel/sacral, solar plexus

Cosmetic Use: N/A

Source and Parts Used: leaves and stems of the aromatic plant

Caution: *Individuals on blood thinners should avoid dermal use of oregano essential oil. Oregano essential oil is potent and can cause intense burning if misused- do not apply on any part of the body except neat on the soles of the feet. Do not ingest. Do not use long-term; it is a powerful substance for the liver to metabolize, and long-term use could cause unwanted changes in liver function. Avoid vapors and keep away from mucus membranes. Do not overuse- 1 or 2 drops go a very long way and all that is needed.*

Tip: Oregano essential oil kills most microbes, and unlike pharmaceutical antibiotics, microbes do not develop resistance against the potent properties of this oil. *Oregano possesses the most potent antimicrobial properties of all essential oils.* Oil of oregano *supplements* can be purchased in health food stores and are wonderful if ingestion is preferred. Again, like dermal use, do not take the supplement for long periods of time.

Palmarosa (Cymbopogon martinii)

Scent: herbaceous with citrus and rose-like undertones

Clinical Uses: sciatica / neuralgia / cystitis / fungal infections / balancing the cardiovascular system / nervous exhaustion

Body Systems Affected: immune, nervous, urinary, circulatory

Inhalation Effect: calms heart palpitations and anxiety / eases emotional and physical exhaustion

Dermal Effect: may be helpful for sciatica and neuralgia when diluted and used in massage / helpful for bladder infections when diluted and applied to the lower back or applied neat to the soles of the feet / combats fungal infections when applied neat to the soles of the feet / may be helpful for rebounding from nervous exhaustion

Practical Uses: tick repellant / fragrant household cleaner

Vibrational Influence: strengthens and expands the human energy field

Emotional Influence: encourages us to be gentle with ourselves and feel more secure in our own skins and about the journey of life / inspires adaptability / calms jealousy / calms the nerves

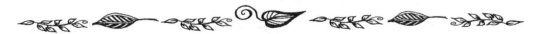

Synergistic to: lemongrass, basil, lavender

Chakra Correspondence: root, navel/sacral

Cosmetic Use: helpful for acne

Source and Parts Used: leaves of the fragrant grass

Caution: *Palmarosa essential oil can cause skin sensitivity if it is applied prior to direct sun exposure or tanning beds. Please wait 24-48 hours before skin is exposed to sunlight or tanning beds. Individuals on blood thinners should avoid dermal use of palmarosa essential oil.*

Palo Santo (Bursera graveolens)

Scent: woody and sweet

Clinical Uses: pain-relief / respiratory ailments / immune support

Body Systems Affected: immune, musculoskeletal, respiratory

Inhalation Effect: deepens and frees up the breath / sharpens the thought process while calming the nerves

Dermal Effect: boosts the immune system / eases muscle and joint pain / may be helpful for respiratory conditions of bacterial or viral origin

Practical Uses: makes a fragrant room spray to clean the air both physically and energetically

Vibrational Influence: carries the energy of protection / raises frequency of the body / integrates emotions and experiences / cleanses the energy field of people and places

Emotional Influence: calms the mind when thoughts, over-analysis, and emotions become obsessive / reduces anxiety, especially mental

Synergistic to: Atlas cedarwood, frankincense, myrrh

Chakra Correspondence: all

Cosmetic Use: a few drops added to distilled water or rose water and added to a spray bottle makes a wonderful spritzer for body and spirit

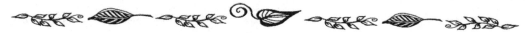

Source and Parts Used: heartwood from the aged, fallen tree

Tip: The palo santo tree is also called holy wood.

Patchouli (Pogostemon patchouli)

Scent: freshly-turned soil, woody with herbaceous undertones

Clinical Uses: premenstrual syndrome (PMS) / nervousness / diarrhea or constipation / excessive perspiration / symptoms of mild depression

Body Systems Affected: reproductive, nervous, gastrointestinal, integumentary

Inhalation Effect: uplifts the mood and quells discontent / calms the nerves

Dermal Effect: helpful for water retention, moodiness, and intestinal upset associated with female hormonal swings, PMS, and perimenopause / very effective in stopping diarrhea (viral) when diluted and combined with 1 drop of sweet orange and clove essential oils and applied to the abdomen 2x a day

Practical Uses: nice scent to use for clothes when sprinkled generously onto a damp wash cloth and added with wet clothes in the dryer / makes an inviting room spray when combined with sweet orange or clove

Vibrational Influence: invites contentment, abundance, and nourishment on the spiritual and emotional levels

Emotional Influence: instills a sense of stability, self-reliance, and calm / helpful in easing symptoms of mild depression and circumstantial depression

Synergistic to: vetiver, geranium

Chakra Correspondence: root, navel/sacral, solar plexus

Cosmetic Use: makes an effective deodorant when sprinkled into distilled water and sprayed on the body / used in numerous cosmetics and as a base note-fixative in perfumery / helpful for reducing the appearance of cellulite when diluted and used in massage

Source and Parts Used: from the slightly-fermented leaves of the plant

Tip: patchouli's aroma deepens beautifully with age, and some suppliers carry aged patchouli essential oil specifically for perfumery

Peppermint (Mentha piperata)

Scent: strong, cool mint

Clinical Uses: irritable bowel syndrome (IBS) / digestive upsets of all kinds / liver and gallbladder support / colds and flu / weak immunity / viral and bacterial infections / lethargy and everyday tiredness / fevers / hot flashes from female hormonal shifts / heat stroke / sinus and lung congestion / sinus pain / chemical and food sensitivities / allergies and hay fever / musculoskeletal, menstrual, and intestinal spasms / spasms of smooth muscles / arthritis / rheumatoid arthritis / mild-moderate depression / hepatitis / colitis / sinus headaches / tension headaches / migraine headaches / poor concentration / Chronis Fatigue Syndrome (Myalgic Encephalomyelitis) / poor circulation / acute and chronic stress / fibromyalgia and other chronic pain syndromes / menstrual cramps / systemic inflammation / systemic candida / low blood pressure

Body Systems Affected: gastrointestinal, immune, endocrine, respiratory, nervous, musculoskeletal, circulatory

Inhalation Effect: can be diffused into the air via nebulizer to combat bacteria, viruses, and molds, especially useful to clear the air of sickrooms / relieves sinus congestion and opens up bronchial passages / uplifts mood and has antidepressant properties / reduces sinus pain when inhaled in a steam (no more than 1 or 2 drops in hot water; avoid steam getting into eyes) / boosts energy levels and useful for general fatigue, rainy day sleepiness, and apathy / helpful as a study aid to sharpen memory, keep the mind alert, and increase concentration; inhale for 5 minutes or so before taking exams / restores a tired nervous system

Dermal Effect: greatly improves circulation when applied neat to the soles of the feet (2-3 drops per sole of the foot) or diluted and used in Swedish massage / cools the body during hot weather when applied neat to the soles of the feet or 1 drop to the palms of the hands; *in cases of heat exhaustion or heat stroke, apply to the soles of the feet as soon as possible*

and use cool compress dipped in peppermint water and place on forehead (add 2 drops of peppermint essential oil to a bowl of cool water, swish around and then dip in a washcloth or hand towel) / apply neat to the soles of the feet to boost immunity for flus, colds, and infections / dilute and apply to abdomen and lower back for menstrual cramps / dilute and apply to sore muscles, arthritis, and soft-tissue injuries / apply neat to the soles of the feet to support the liver and gallbladder and improve function of both organs / apply neat to the soles of the feet for systemic candida or yeast overgrowth in the intestines / apply neat to the soles of the feet to decrease frequency and intensity of hot flashes during menopause / apply neat to the soles of the feet for seasonal allergies and chemical, environmental, and food sensitivities; especially effective when used after ingestion of dairy and exposure to pollens and molds / apply neat to the soles of the feet or use diluted in massage to decrease systemic inflammation / apply neat to the soles of the feet, use diluted in massage, footbath, or bath to restore and soothe the nervous system / apply neat to soles of the feet and apply cool compress dipped in peppermint water and place on forehead to break an adult fever that is too high *(add 2 drops of peppermint essential oil to a bowl of cool water, swish around and then dip in a washcloth or hand towel)* / apply cool compress dipped in peppermint water and place on forehead for tension headache or migraine if the aroma is tolerated *(add 2 drops of peppermint essential oil to a bowl of cool water, swish around and then dip in a washcloth or hand towel)* / excellent for intestinal distress, colitis, and griping pain when diluted and applied to abdomen up to 3x a day / apply neat to the soles of the feet to boost blood pressure

Practical Uses: Peppermint essential oil can be applied neat to the soles of the feet in the morning to help the body remain cool on hot, summer days / a few drops applied neat to the soles of the feet before traveling will improve circulation during long plane flights or car rides and prevent leg swelling / 1 or 2 drops added to warm water makes an effective mouthwash / nice scent to use for clothes when sprinkled generously onto a damp wash cloth and added with wet clothes in the dryer / a solution of peppermint, water, and borax will eliminate mold / the essential oil will deter spiders, ants, and other insects from entering the home when sprinkled generously along window sills and doors / household cleaner and deodorizing room spray / a speck of peppermint essential oil under the tongue will decrease nausea within minutes or even seconds (touching the point of a wooden toothpick on the bottle of essential oil equals the appropriate amount) / a few drops mixed well into cornstarch and stored in

a grated cheese shaker makes a wonderful, deodorizing foot powder that can be sprinkled into shoes before putting them on

Vibrational Influence: holds the green essence of the natural world and fills energy fields of people and places with vibrant, clean, and invigorating vitality / peppermint essential oil is equal to negative ions present near moving water and the electrical charge in the air after a thunderstorm / excellent oil for caregivers, nurses, doctors, social workers, holistic practitioners, and empaths to cleanse accumulated energy and emotions absorbed from other people

Emotional Influence: uplifting to the mind and emotions / dispels apathy and symptoms of depression / renews optimism / inspires enthusiasm

Synergistic to: spearmint, lavender, balsam fir, pine needle, lemongrass

Chakra Correspondence: root, solar plexus, brow

Cosmetic Use: used in numerous cleansers, soaps, shampoos, and cosmetics / excellent, refreshing oil for oily skin and hair—a small amount (a drop or two) can be added to unscented liquid castile soap, shampoo, or hand soap, especially fragrant and antibacterial when combined with lemongrass

Source and Parts Used: leaves and stems from the aromatic plant

Caution: *Peppermint essential oil should not be used on children or infants, however, if is safe to diffuse into the air via nebulizer for short periods of time. Although peppermint is a valuable oil to use in cases of adult fevers when the temperature is high, it is too strong of an oil to use on children and babies; lavender is a wonderful substitution for a child or infant. Peppermint should never be used on pregnant women. Peppermint should not be used excessively by individuals with high blood pressure. Do not apply to cuts, wounds, or broken skin. It should not be used less than 2 hours between homeopathic remedies. Keep away from eyes and mucus membranes.*

Notes: Peppermint essential oil is an adaptogen- stimulating *or* sedating, depending upon the body's needs at the time. It is also an ally in combating E.coli, Strep, Staph, and tuberculosis as well as other viral and bacterial infections.

Peru Balsam (Myroxylon Pereira)

a.k.a. Balsam de Peru

Scent: earthy with deep vanilla undertones

Clinical Uses: lung congestion / eczema

Body Systems Affected: integumentary, respiratory, nervous

Inhalation Effect: breaks up mucus congestion of lungs and sinus / calms the nerves

Dermal Effect: speeds of healing of cuts and skin conditions / stimulates production of new skin

Practical Uses: can be rubbed neat onto candles for a lovely scent; wait at least 4 hours before burning.

Vibrational Influence: inspires peace and empathy for others and oneself

Emotional Influence: inspires a feeling of warm contentment and safety / encourages self-care, self-love / a nice oil for women who forget to pamper themselves every now and then

Synergistic to: benzoin, vanilla

Chakra Correspondence: heart

Cosmetic Use: a drop or two added to natural unscented lotion soothes dry skin

Source and Parts Used: resin from the tree

Caution: *though Peru balsam is good for dry skin, some individuals with very sensitive skin may find it irritating.*

Tip: Peru balsam makes a beautiful perfume by itself that is reminiscent of true amber and can be used to make an amber-like blend by combining it with benzoin and a bit of ylang ylang

Petitgrain (Citrus aurantifolia)

Scent: floral-citrus with woody undertones

Clinical Uses: stress-related conditions / insomnia / indigestion

Body Systems Affected: nervous, gastrointestinal

Inhalation Effect: calms the nerves and prepares the body for sleep / sharpens the mind and improves concentration

Dermal Effect: relieves flatulence and indigestion when diluted and applied to the abdomen / helps the nervous system find balance

Practical Uses: used in household cleaners and fragrant room sprays

Vibrational Influence: carries the energy of stability and compassion for self and others

Emotional Influence: inspires confidence / offers comfort and hope during times of vulnerability

Synergistic to: neroli, sweet orange

Chakra Correspondence: solar plexus

Cosmetic Use: often substituted for more expensive neroli and used in perfumery

Source and Parts Used: twigs and leaves of the orange tree, most often of the bitter orange also called Seville

Tip: According to some sources, petitgrain essential oil, though sourced from the leaves and twigs of the orange tree, does not cause photosensitivity. However, use with caution in direct sunlight and tanning beds to be safe.

Pine Bark (Pinus sylvestris)

Scent: deep, pungent pine with woody and root-like overtones

Clinical Uses: adrenal and kidney support / chronic stress / weak immunity / exhaustion from stress / multiple sclerosis / general endocrine support

Body Systems Affected: endocrine, respiratory, nervous, urinary

Inhalation Effect: encourages stability, practicality, and self-reliance

Dermal Effect: helps support the adrenals when applied neat to the soles of the feet / strengthens the kidneys and bladder when applied neat to the soles of the feet / apply neat to the soles of the feet or diluted and used in Swedish massage during times of low energy reserves / may be helpful for symptoms of multiple sclerosis (MS) / good oil during flu season when diluted and rubbed onto the chest for coughs and colds / promotes balance to the entire endocrine system when applied neat to the soles of the feet or diluted and used in massage / excellent for non-Addison's adrenal exhaustion especially when combined with frankincense and balsam fir and applied neat upon rising and before bed, or diluted and used in massage / boosts immunity when combined with clove essential oil and applied neat to the soles of the feet

Practical Uses: added to household cleaners

Vibrational Influence: provides grounding and a sense of security / encourages willingness to survive extreme emotional, mental, physical, and spiritual adversity

Emotional Influence: helps us to remember our own strength / give us a boost of energy when our reserves are running low

Synergistic to: juniper berry, cypress

Chakra Correspondence: root, solar plexus

Cosmetic Use: can be added to shampoo to control dry, flaky scalp and dandruff

Source and Parts Used: bark of the tree

Tip: Be sure to not confuse pine bark essential oil with *pine needle essential oil*; both are from the same tree but offer benefits that are unique.

<u>Pine Needle</u> (Pinus sylvestris)

Scent: soft evergreen, like the crushed needles

Clinical Uses: muscle and joint pain / bronchitis / low energy / kidney and bladder support

Body Systems Affected: musculoskeletal, respiratory, endocrine, urinary

Inhalation Effect: eases sinus pressure and pain during colds and flu, especially when used in a steam / decreases moodiness / promotes clarity of thought and readiness to get things done

Dermal Effect: decreases muscle and joint pain, especially when combined with eucalyptus, peppermint, or ginger essential oil / excellent for urinary tract infections when diluted and applied to the lower back, kidney area, and the abdomen / relieves everyday fatigue when applied neat to the soles of the feet in the morning / has restoring effect on the nervous system / soothing to the body in cases of colds and flus and beneficial to the immune system when diluted and applied all over the body / helps sooth coughs and bronchitis when diluted and applied to the chest and throat

Practical Uses: used in household cleaners, room sprays, and air fresheners / invites peaceful sleep when sprinkled onto sheets and blankets before bed

Vibrational Influence: invites new energies, plans, and beginnings / holds the green soul-energy of the natural world / expands the human energy field / clears away dark thoughts, pessimism, and emotional heaviness

Emotional Influence: helps to lift emotional burdens and misplaced guilt / promotes self-preservation and self-care / decreases symptoms of depression / lessens excessive, obsessive worry about the future and the wellbeing of others

Synergistic to: black spruce, balsam fir, peppermint

Chakra Correspondence: root, solar plexus

Cosmetic Use: used in soaps and perfumery

Source and Parts Used: needles (leaves) of the tree

Plai (Zingiber cassumunar)

Scent: pungent and bright with black pepper and eucalyptus-like undertones

Clinical Uses: severe asthma / muscle and joint pain / rheumatoid arthritis and other chronic pain syndromes / poor circulation / post-operative pain / pain from irritable bowel syndrome (IBS) / menstrual pain / inflammation

Body Systems Affected: respiratory, musculoskeletal, circulatory, nervous

Inhalation Effect: may reduce asthma attacks in some individuals when diffused into the air via nebulizer

Dermal Effect: may reduce asthma attacks in some individuals when diluted and applied to the chest / has been shown to reduce pain after surgery and lessen the need for pain killers / improves circulation when applied neat to the soles of the feet or diluted and used in massage / reduces pain when diluted and rubbed into muscles and joints / reduces menstrual pain when diluted and applied to abdomen and lower back / reduces pain from irritable bowel syndrome when diluted and applied to abdomen, especially the lower belly / reduces systemic inflammation when diluted and used in massage or applied neat to the soles of the feet

Practical Uses: added to refreshing room sprays and air fresheners

Vibrational Influence: raises the frequency of places and people

Emotional Influence: brightens the mood

Synergistic to: ginger, helichrysum

Chakra Correspondence: root, navel/sacral, heart

Cosmetic Use: N/A

Source and Parts Used: rhizomes of the plant

Ravensara (Ravensara aromatica)

a.k.a. Agathophyllum aromatica

Scent: sweetly herbaceous with subtle anise-like undertones

Clinical Uses: viral infections / chicken pox and shingles / weak immunity / skin healing / post-shingles neuralgia / influenza

Body Systems Affected: respiratory, immune

Inhalation Effect: may be helpful for stubborn sinus infections when used in a steam and inhaled 1-2x daily / uplifts the mood

Dermal Effect: excellent to combat chicken pox and shingles when applied neat to the soles of the feet and diluted and applied along the spine / can be diluted and applied directly to chicken pox or shingles rash to decrease discomfort and speed healing; nourishes the nerves and may prevent the risk of developing post-shingles neuralgia / applied neat to the soles of the feet for more severe bouts of the flu or applied while in good health to boost immunity during the flu season

Practical Uses: household cleaner

Vibrational Influence: sweeps away low-frequency energies and emotions from places, especially where heated emotions have built up over time

Emotional Influence: improves mood, especially useful for afternoon slumps

Synergistic to: helichrysum, geranium, Australian blue cypress, lavender

Chakra Correspondence: root

Cosmetic Use: used in lotions and applications for troubled, inflamed skin

Source and Parts Used: leaves of the tree

Tip: Do not confuse ravensara essential with *ravintsara* essential oil, two distinctly different sources.

Ravintsara (Cinnamomum camphora)

Scent: eucalyptus-like with cinnamon overtones

Clinical Uses: viral infections and prevention of viral replication / shingles / sinus infection / respiratory support

Body Systems Affected: respiratory, immune

Inhalation Effect: combats viruses and keeps healthy people well when diffused into the air via nebulizer / helpful for sinus infections

Dermal Effect: apply neat to the soles of the feet to boost immunity, especially to prevent and diminish viral attacks / dilute and apply to the chest for lung infections, flu, and colds / dilute in tamanu carrier oil and apply to shingles rash for quicker healing process and less discomfort Tip:

Tamanu oil is a skin-nourishing oil that possesses antibacterial properties and makes an excellent carrier oil for immune-boosting essential oils

Practical Uses: effective household cleaner

Vibrational Influence: cleanses and strengthens the energy field

Emotional Influence: N/A

Synergistic to: eucalyptus radiata, tea tree, niaouli

Chakra Correspondence: root, heart

Cosmetic Use: N/A

Source and Parts Used: leaves of the tree

Tip: Ravintsara essential oil can be substituted for eucalyptus essential oil

<u>Rosalina</u> (Melaleuca ericifolia)

a.k.a. Lavender Tea Tree

Scent: similar to tea tree but softer

Clinical Uses: viral, bacterial, and fungal infections / children's head colds / acne /

Body Systems Affected: immune, respiratory, nervous

Inhalation Effect: effective for sinus infections / calms the nerves

Dermal Effect: combats all types of infections when applied neat to the soles of the feet / antiseptic and nourishing for skin troubled by acne; can be applied neat onto pimples (if skin is sensitive, dilute with distilled or tap water and use as a skin spritzer)

Practical Uses: combats respiratory infections when diffused into the air via nebulizer

Vibrational Influence: clears away dark thoughts and emotions from places and people

Emotional Influence: encourages a sense of stability and grounding during transitional or emotional times

Synergistic to: tea tree, eucalyptus

Chakra Correspondence: root

Cosmetic Use: can be used in cleansers and skin spritzers for acne

Source and Parts Used: leaves of the tree

Tip: Rosalina essential oil is a wonderful oil for children and anyone who prefers a softer scent than pungent tea tree essential oil. Rosalina is a cousin of the tea tree and is known to be as effective.

Rose (Rosa damascene, Rosa centifolia)

a.k.a. Rose Otto and Rose Absolute

Scent: like the flower, some varieties sweeter than others

Clinical Uses: hormonal and nervous system imbalances / symptoms of mild-moderate depression / dopamine production in the brain / homeostasis of the body

Body Systems Affected: nervous, reproductive, dermal

Inhalation Effect: releases endorphins—namely dopamine—the neurotransmitter released by the brain in copious amounts when we are in love and feeling euphoric / eases depression, anxiety, and feelings of dread / may increase tolerance for pain and useful to inhale before dental or other procedures / improves orgasmic response in women and increases semen in men <u>Tip:</u> the best and most economical way to use rose as an inhalation oil is to put a drop or two on a tissue or in an aroma locket

Dermal Effect: brings balance to the entire body by promoting homeostasis within the nervous system / like the herb, may boost immune response

Practical Uses: can be inhaled for 10-15 minutes before dental and other procedures to ease nerves and increase tolerance to pain

Vibrational Influence: restores people and places to a state of harmony / invites energies of highest frequency

Emotional Influence: soothes a heart broken from grief, loss, or change / promotes love in all forms, including spiritual love and respect for self / eases symptoms of depression and offers new perspective even in hopeless situations

Synergistic to: cacao, ylang ylang, neroli

Chakra Correspondence: navel/sacral, solar plexus, heart, high heart, crown

Cosmetic Use: used in numerous cosmetics and perfumery / balances and nourishes all skin types when added to beauty oils and lotions / a few drops, even the diluted form added to distilled water or culinary rosewater makes a fragrant face and body spritzer to apply before make-up or used as cooling spray when put into the fridge before use

Source and Parts Used: whole flowers

Tip: Rose otto, from the Damask rose, is considered to be a superior oil for clinical and therapeutic applications. Rose possesses the highest frequency of all essential oils and a drop or two combined with other oils will raise the frequency of the others. Creating synergistic blends with a little rose added can make them more effective on the physical, emotional, and vibrational levels. For a nourishing and lovely face spritzer for all skin types, combine a few drops of diluted rose otto or absolute with diluted Roman chamomile to distilled water in a spray bottle—shake before each use.

Notes: 250 or more varieties of rose exist as well as 10,000 hybrids. Rose essential oils differ in their scents, and the Bulgarian variety is considered the most sought-after in the world of perfumery. Despite their differences, all rose essential oils have significant uses in clinical aromatherapy. Rose absolute and rose otto essential oils are one of the most costly but are available in diluted form and quite affordable; diluted rose possesses all of the unique properties of the concentrated. It is estimated that 60 roses are needed to make a single drop of undiluted rose absolute, hence the high cost of this lovely essence.

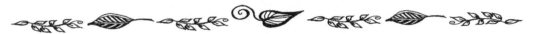

Rosehip (Rosa canina)
a.k.a. as Rosa mosqueta

Scent: nutty and mild

Clinical Uses: sun damage to the skin / scars / psoriasis / eczema

Body Systems Affected: integumentary

Inhalation Effect: N/A

Dermal Effect: when used consistently, highly effective in diminishing age spots; apply daily for 4 months; may be combined with frankincense for added benefits / regenerates skin damaged by the sun, radiation treatments, and the natural aging process / reduces scars, especially surgical scars / effective for stubborn, chronic eczema, and psoriasis

Practical Uses: N/A

Vibrational Influence: N/A

Emotional Influence: N/A

Synergistic to: sea buckthorn, frankincense

Chakra Correspondence: heart

Cosmetic Use: used in numerous skin preparations

Source and Parts Used: from the seeds and sometimes also the whole fruit of the rose

Tip: Apply neat or added to natural moisturizer or carrier oil. Rosehip essential oil's profound skin benefits are due to its high content of essential fatty acids (EFAs); rosehip essential oil consists of 77% EFAs and is high in natural retinol, linolenic acids, and vitamin C. Due to its high content of fatty acids, rosehip essential oil is not recommended for oily or acne-prone skin.

Rosemary (Rosmarinus officinalis)

Scent: green and herbaceous, pungent

Clinical Uses: afternoon fatigue / poor memory / multiple sclerosis / sinus congestion

Body Systems Affected: endocrine, nervous, respiratory

Inhalation Effect: helpful for sinus pain from allergies and colds; best used in a steam / uplifts the spirit and decreases apathy / restorative effect on the mind exhausted from work, studying, or worry / provides the body with a boost of energy during long work days or afternoon slumps / improves memory and may be helpful to inhale before taking exams / <u>Tip:</u> for mood enhancement, afternoon tiredness, and memory, 1 drop on a tissue or in an aroma locket is the best method of inhalation

Dermal Effect: may be effective for symptoms of multiple sclerosis (MS) when diluted and used in massage (only 1 drop per session)

Practical Uses: household cleaner, room sprays, and air freshener

Vibrational Influence: cleans the energy field of people and places, and charges the environment with vitality of the natural world

Emotional Influence: offers invigorating energy, lifting burdens of the heart and psyche

Synergistic to: basil, peppermint

Chakra Correspondence: root, solar plexus, heart, high heart, brow

Cosmetic Use: may be helpful for alopecia when diluted and rubbed into the scalp

Source and Parts Used: "leaves" and stems of the aromatic plant

Caution: *Rosemary should not be used by anyone with, epilepsy or any predisposition to seizures. Individuals with moderate-severe reactive/non-diabetic hypoglycemia (low blood sugar) should use rosemary sparingly. It is an oil that should be used minimally in dermal use; according to some sources, it can build up over time in the blood and be toxic. Non-excessive inhalation is okay.*

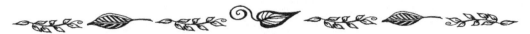

Rosewood (Aniba rosaeodora)

a.k.a. Bois de Rose

Scent: rose-like with woody and citrus undertones

Clinical Uses: systemic candida / shingles / acute grief / adrenal support / nervous exhaustion / overall toning and balance of the body's organ systems / insomnia / emotional exhaustion with physical symptoms of burnout / headaches accompanied by nausea / immune support / skin regeneration

Body Systems Affected: immune, nervous, integumentary, endocrine

Inhalation Effect: eases symptoms of depression and deep sadness / supports the nervous system and adrenals during times of stress, especially emotional / calms the mind and eases anxiety / promotes deep sleep, especially when combined with neroli, lavender, and/or ylang ylang

Dermal Effect: strengthens the body's immune defense / promotes equilibrium of the body's systems / tones the nervous system, balancing extremes / supports the adrenals during times of stress, especially when diluted and used in Swedish massage and applied along the spine / promotes sleep and combats insomnia when applied neat to the soles of the feet / excellent oil to use for migraines and other headaches accompanied by nausea, provided the scent is tolerated; dilute and apply all over the body or neat to the soles of the feet / combats systemic and intestinal candida albicans when applied neat to the soles of the feet / For general nervous debility, rosewood works extremely well with frankincense and lavender when applied neat to the soles of the feet and diluted and used in massage

Practical Uses: can be applied neat to the soles of the feet and inhaled to rebound from jetlag

Vibrational Influence: bathes people and places with soothing, maternal energy

Emotional Influence: unsurpassed for comforting a heart broken by grief, loss, transition, and emotional exhaustion / highly effective for acute grief when combined with sandalwood / can be combined with ylang ylang to calm the body and mind after intense emotions and arguments / lifts depression / best used in Swedish massage and aroma locket

Synergistic to: frankincense, ylang ylang, lavender, ravensara

Chakra Correspondence: root, heart, high heart

Cosmetic Use: used in lotions and oils to rejuvenate the skin

Source and Parts Used: wood from the tree

Tip: *Rosewood essential oil may be applied neat in small amounts. Rosewood trees are highly endangered trees due to rain forest deterioration. You may consider purchasing this oil from companies that are conscious of this situation and harvest from specified sources.*

<u>Sage</u> (Salvia officinalis)

Scent: green and herbaceous, pungent

Clinical Uses: mental and physical fatigue

Body Systems Affected: nervous, respiratory

Inhalation Effect: a drop or two added to a steam opens sinuses / sharpens the mind for mental work / uplifts the mood / gives the body a boost of energy when needed

Dermal Effect: N/A

Practical Uses: nice scent to use for clothes when sprinkled generously with Texas cedar onto a damp wash cloth and added with wet clothes in the dryer / 1 drop combined with one drop of Texas cedar on a hairbrush will give hair a pleasant woody-grassy scent / makes an invigorating room spray and air freshener

Vibrational Influence: clears away psychic and emotional debris when used in a room spritzer or diffused into the air via nebulizer / defends against low-frequency energies

Emotional Influence: lifts dark moods and feelings of boredom

Synergistic to: Texas cedar, juniper berry

Chakra Correspondence: root, brow, crown

Cosmetic Use: N/A

172

Source and Parts Used: the leaves of the plant known as common sage a.k.a. Dalmatian sage

Caution: *Not recommended for dermal use due to its high content of ketones which can be toxic. Individuals with epilepsy or seizure disorders should not use sage essential oil. Avoid inhaling during pregnancy. Do not inhale excessively.*

Tip: Do not confuse sage essential oil with *clary sage* essential oil; unlike sage, clary sage *(Salvia sclarea)* is the only sage considered appropriate for dermal use.

Sandalwood (Santalum album)

a.k.a. Indian Sandalwood

Scent: sweet and woody

Clinical Uses: cystitis / restlessness, insomnia, and disturbed sleep / hypoxia (low oxygen levels) / autism / acute grief / anxiety and nervousness / skin cancer prevention / fungal skin infections / immune support

Body Systems Affected: nervous, urinary, circulatory, respiratory

Inhalation Effect: greatly increases oxygen levels in the brain and bodily tissues / decreases anxiety and lifts depression / comforts a heart burdened with grief / directly affects the pineal gland, therefore excellent for promoting relaxation during meditation

Dermal Effect: applied to the soles of the feet combats urinary tract infections / brings balance to the nervous system / promotes undisturbed sleep / may be helpful in preventing skin cancer caused by chemical exposure and UV rays / combats fungal infections of nail beds and skin / can be diluted and applied to the chest and throat for respiratory infections

Practical Uses: N/A

Vibrational Influence: integrates the physical and the spiritual / eases transitions, including death and the death of a loved one

Emotional Influence: offers comfort and grounding during acute grief / excellent oil to use in hospice work

Synergistic to: frankincense, palo santo

Chakra Correspondence: all

Cosmetic Use: used in numerous cosmetics, lotions, and preparations to revitalize, balance, and nourish the skin / good for all skin types, especially mature skin

Source and Parts Used: heartwood of the tree

Tip: *Please note that sandalwood trees must live a long time before their heartwood can be used and their oil extracted/distilled. Due to commercial exploitation, these trees are now endangered. With environmental awareness, some aromatherapists choose not to use Indian sandalwood oil at all; yet some use it sparingly because many believe that its properties cannot be fully substituted. There are other wonderful types of sandalwood available, including: <u>Australian Sandalwood</u> (Santalum spicatum), <u>New Caledonia Sandalwood</u> (Santalum austrocaledonium), and <u>Royal Hawaiian Sandalwood</u> (Santalum paniculatum). Sandalwood essential oil is available in diluted form and contains its beneficial properties, but for combating bladder and other infections, undiluted sandalwood essential oil is recommended.*

<u>Sea Buckthorn</u> (Hippophae rhamnoides)

Scent: herbaceous with sweet undertones

Clinical Uses: healing of skin conditions / alopecia / bed sores

Body Systems Affected: integumentary

Inhalation Effect: N/A

Dermal Effect: excellent for all skin conditions including dermatitis, eczema, burns, cuts, burns from x-rays and radiation, bed sores, skin ulcers, and changes in skin pigment / may stimulate hair growth in cases of alopecia when diluted and rubbed into the scalp

Practical Uses: N/A

Vibrational Influence: N/A

Emotional Influence: N/A

Synergistic to: carrot seed, rosehip, helichrysum

Chakra Correspondence: N/A

Cosmetic Use: used in numerous cosmetics and anti-aging skin preparations

Source and Parts Used: berries from the plant

Caution: *Sea buckthorn is available as an herbal supplement and recommended for many conditions; however, the herb is contraindicated for individuals on blood thinners, including aspirin.*

Tip: Sea Buckthorn essential oil is deep orange in color and can stain clothing; it may initially leave an orange hue on the skin until absorbed.

Spearmint (Mentha spicata)

Scent: sweet mint, milder and softer than peppermint

Clinical Uses: digestive upset and nausea / muscle sprains, strains, and pain / gout / female hormonal balance / symptoms of mild-moderate depression / muscle spasms / menstrual cramps / menstrual headaches / tension headaches / morning tiredness / oral health / children's aches and pains / poor memory / intestinal discomfort from constipation or diarrhea

Body Systems Affected: gastrointestinal, musculoskeletal, endocrine

Inhalation Effect: brightens the spirits / calms the nerves / sharpens the mind and memory / excellent study aid if inhaled on a tissue 5 minutes before taking exams / 1 undiluted drop on the palms of the hands and inhaled decreases nausea and queasiness; the same amount can also be applied to a tissue and inhaled / helps to relieves sinus pain and congestion from allergies and colds when added with other essential oils to a steam / can be applied generously to a damp or wet wash cloth or towel and placed into a sauna / wakes up the body on tired and sluggish mornings / good oil to inhale at work or school during afternoon slumps

Dermal Effect: 1 drop diluted and applied to the chest eases coughs and congestion in non-asthmatic children and adults (do not use under the age of 5) / 1 or 2 drops diluted and added to unscented lotion or carrier oil can be applied to sore muscles and joints to lessen pain and have an

antiflammatory effect / very useful to prevent or decrease post-workout muscle soreness and recommended for sports massage / helps to balance the female hormonal system when applied to the soles of the feet; especially useful in easing physical symptoms of premenstrual syndrome (PMS) including menstrual headache—for best results, use 3-4x during the week leading up to the menstrual period and give it 2-3 months to see significant results; can be applied neat to the feet for menstrual headaches, water retention, and queasy hormonal bellies / can be diluted and applied on the abdomen for after-eating bloating or hormone-related distention, intestinal rumbling or diarrhea / can be double diluted and applied to the abdomen for children's stomach aches / dilute and apply to the neck and shoulders for tension headaches / has a gentle restorative effect on the nervous system

Practical Uses: insect repellant / 1 drop added to warm water, especially when combined with lemongrass, makes a pleasant and effective mouthwash / a speck on the tip of a wooden toothpick and applied under the tongue will dramatically decrease nausea or belching, especially during women's hormonal swings; can be applied up to 4x an hour / makes a delightful household cleaner, room spray, and air freshener especially when combined with lavender

Vibrational Influence: sweeps people and places with invigorating newness / a good oil to spray when moving into a new living or work space

Emotional Influence: lifts the spirits and balances emotional extremes

Synergistic to: peppermint, basil

Chakra Correspondence: navel/sacral, solar plexus

Cosmetic Use: small amounts can be added to cleanser and shower gel for toning the skin / good for oily *non-inflamed* skin

Source and Parts Used: leaves and stems of the aromatic plant

Caution: *Do not apply to cuts or open skin. Keep away from mucus membranes of eyes, nose, undiluted in the mouth, and the genital area.*

Tip: Spearmint essential oil shares many of the same properties as peppermint, but it is unique in its ability to balance female hormones. It also has a warming action whereas peppermint has a cooling effect on the muscles and the body in general. A little goes a long way. For symptoms of

perimenopause and menopause, combining spearmint with clary sage essential oil may be helpful.

Spikenard (Nardostachys jatamansi)

Scent: valerian-like, musty

Clinical Uses: nervous conditions / stubborn, relentless skin rashes especially of nervous origin / allergic skin reactions / anxiety and panic attacks / nightmares and fears that disrupt sleep / addiction recovery / heart support / dandruff

Body Systems Affected: nervous, integumentary

Inhalation Effect: helps recovery from addiction / calms heart palpitations from nervous origin

Dermal Effect: excellent essential oil for insomnia when applied to the soles of the feet; its deep sedative properties are enhanced for this purpose when combined with Atlas cedarwood and rosewood / helps recovery from addiction when used with massage and combined with lavender, rose, and ylang ylang / calms heart palpitations from nervous origin when used in Swedish massage / reduces deep-seated anxiety when applied neat to the soles of the feet, especially combined with ylang ylang, lavender, or neroli / effective for relentless skin rashes and a good oil to try when all else fails / helps the skin to heal and the cells to rejuvenate

Practical Uses: N/A

Vibrational Influence: carries the energy of deep, uncompromised peace / promotes inner stillness and spiritual quests

Emotional Influence: instills peace / helps recovery from addiction

Synergistic to: Atlas cedarwood, frankincense, rosewood, myrrh

Chakra Correspondence: solar plexus, heart

Cosmetic Use: effective for dandruff when diluted and applied to the scalp, conditioner, and shampoo; use juniper berry, patchouli, and ylang ylang essential oils for enhanced effectiveness and pleasant scent

Source and Parts Used: rhizomes and roots of the aromatic plant

Tip: Spikenard is related to valerian and has a musty scent that is best blended with other oils to bring out its more pleasant undertones. A little goes a long way. Like sandalwood and cassia essential oil, the aroma of spikenard improves and deepens with age. It is associated with Mary Magdalene.

Spruce, Black (Picea mariana)

Scent: deep forest evergreen with sweet undertones

Clinical Uses: hyperthyroidism / excessive cortisol production / chronic stress / adrenal support / general endocrine balance / Chronic Fatigue Syndrome (CFS) / fibromyalgia / lung support / coughs

Body Systems Affected: endocrine, respiratory

Inhalation Effect: acts as a decongestant and supports the lungs when inhaled via steam / improves the mood

Dermal Effect: balances excessive thyroid hormone production when applied neat to the soles of the feet / applied neat to the soles of the feet to minimize excessive cortisol levels in the body / diluted and used in massage modalities to lower the stress response in the body / applied neat to the soles of the feet to promote overall endocrine balance / apply diluted to the kidney area 3-4x a week for adrenal fatigue and to support the adrenals during times of stress / use diluted in massage and apply neat to the soles of the feet for Chronic Fatigue Syndrome and fibromyalgia / can be used in the bath for a restorative effect on the body and psyche

Practical Uses: added to natural potpourri and room sprays to scent the home

Vibrational Influence: increases prana or life force of an individual / holds the "green" vitality of the earth and the natural world

Emotional Influence: lifts despondency

Synergistic to: pine needle, frankincense, lavender, balsam fir

Chakra Correspondence: root, solar plexus

Cosmetic Use: used in perfumes and colognes

Source and Parts Used: needles and twigs of the black spruce tree

Caution: *Spruce essential oil should not be applied prior to exposure to sunlight or tanning beds. Wait 24 hours to be sure.*

Tip: *Black spruce essential oil is highly recommended for those who have an overabundance of stress in their daily lives or who are experiencing burnout.*

<u>Storax</u> (liquidambar orientalis)

Scent: woody and vanilla-like with sweet undertones

Clinical Uses: physical and mental anxiety / emotional exhaustion

Body Systems Affected: nervous/limbic

Inhalation Effect: calms worry, anxiety, and dread

Dermal Effect: N/A

Practical Uses: scenting rooms, especially bedroom and office to induce calm

Vibrational Influence: strengthens energy field / aligns physical body with the spiritual Self / resonates with the mysteries of the Sacred Feminine or Goddess energy

Emotional Influence: instills sense of security / promotes spirituality / helps one to be more comfortable in the physical body and increases tolerance for one's physical health challenges

Synergistic to: benzoin, myrrh, spikenard, frankincense

Chakra Correspondence: all, but a special affinity to the heart, high heart, and crown

Cosmetic Use: ingredient in perfumes

Source and Parts Used: balsam from the wood and inner bark of the tree

179

Tip: Storax is sometimes referred to as "amber." Please bear in mind that almost 100% of the time, fragrance oils labeled "amber" are synthetic or a blend of natural and chemical sources. Please look for amber blends offered by therapeutic-grade companies. Imitations have no therapeutic value. Benzoin (Styrax benzoin) often is a key ingredient in true essential oil blends labeled as "amber." If you'd like to make your own beautiful amber blend, use equal parts benzoin or storax and Peru balsam with a drop or two of ylang ylang.

<u>Tagetes</u> (Tagetes bipinata)

a.k.a. Southern Marigold

Scent: pungent, similar to garden marigolds and chrysanthemums

Clinical Uses: infections of the nail bed / fungal infections in general

Body Systems Affected: dermal, immune

Inhalation Effect: uplifts mood

Dermal Effect: highly effective for fungal nail infections when diluted and applied to the nail bed / combats systemic fungal infections and candida when applied neat to the soles of the feet

Practical Uses: fly and insect repellant

Vibrational Influence: carries protective energy

Emotional Influence: promotes positivity and cheerfulness

Synergistic to: sandalwood, calendula

Chakra Correspondence: solar plexus, heart

Cosmetic Use: used in small amounts in perfumery

Source and Parts Used: flowers of the shrub related to the common marigold

Caution: *Tagetes essential oil should not be applied prior to exposure to sunlight or tanning beds. Wait 24 hours to be sure. Could irritate sensitive skin; in this case, dilute well.*

Tip: Do not confuse tagetes essential oil with calendula (marigold) essential oil.

<u>Tangerine (Citrus reticulata)</u>

Scent: like the fruit, bright citrus with sweet overtones

Clinical Uses: anxiety / children's nervousness and restlessness / supports the adult and juvenile digestive system / stretch marks and cellulite

Body Systems Affected: nervous, gastrointestinal, integumentary

Inhalation Effect: brightens the mood and calms the nerves / inspires happiness

Dermal Effect: promotes peristalsis and effective for adult and children's constipation or diarrhea when diluted and applied to the abdomen / reduces the appearance of cellulite when diluted and massaged into the skin / reduces stretch marks when diluted and massaged into the skin

Practical Uses: lovely when added to household cleaners, room sprays, potpourri, and air fresheners

Vibrational Influence: carries the energy of stability, hope, and joy

Emotional Influence: lifts the mood and calms the nerves in both children and adults

Synergistic to: grapefruit, Roman chamomile

Chakra Correspondence: solar plexus

Cosmetic Use: used in perfumes and fragrant body and hair spritzers

Source and Parts Used: peels of the fruit

Tip: Tangerine essential oil is often bright orange in color and may stain light-colored clothing; to avoid this, apply to skin and hair.

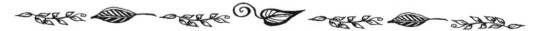

Tarragon (Artemisia dracunculus)

Scent: herbaceous with anise-like undertones

Clinical Uses: menstrual pain / urinary tract infections / intestinal spasms / decreasing uric acid in the body / general muscle spasm and pain / poor circulation of blood and lymph / appetite stimulant

Body Systems Affected: urinary, musculoskeletal

Inhalation Effect: 1 drop on a tissue or in an aroma locket for a calming effect on the nerves or to stimulate appetite

Dermal Effect: a small amount diluted and applied to the abdomen and lower back has a warming, antispasmodic effect for menstrual cramps, muscle spasms, and aches and pains especially when combined with spearmint essential oil / a drop or two diluted and used in Swedish massage will stimulate circulation of both blood and lymph, therefore preventing uric acid from accumulating in the joints / a small amount diluted and applied to the abdomen and the area of the kidneys will ease discomfort of urinary tract infections; for best results, apply sandalwood essential oil neat to the soles of the feet

Practical Uses: insect repellant

Vibrational Influence: N/A

Emotional Influence: calms the nerves while uplifting the mood and boosting mental clarity when inhaled in small amounts

Synergistic to: spearmint, peppermint, anise seed

Chakra Correspondence: navel/sacral, solar plexus

Cosmetic Use: N/A

Source and Parts Used: leaves and flowering tops of the aromatic plant

Caution: *Tarragon essential oil should not be used by individuals with epilepsy or seizure disorders. Do not use on children. Due to its powerful chemistry, use sparingly and not habitually in dermal blends; inhalation is considered okay.*

Notes: Tarragon essential oil has been shown to inhibit the growth of pathogens including Staphylococcus aureus and E.coli and may be developed as a preservative for foods such as cheeses.

Tea Tree (Melaleuca alternifolia)

a.k.a. Melaleuca

Scent: pungent and medicinal

Clinical Uses: all viral, bacterial, and fungal infections / low immunity / systemic candida / Athlete's foot / acne / Epstein-Barr virus and syndrome / Chronic Fatigue Syndrome / allergies / food poisoning / shock / colds and flu / nervous collapse / gingivitis and gum disease / wound healing / warts

Body Systems Affected: immune, integumentary, nervous

Inhalation Effect: combats sinus infections and chronic sinusitis when used in steams

Dermal Effect: combine with lemon, white thyme, clove, or lavender essential oil to boost the immune system, fight infections and the flu / tea tree added to a foot bath will eliminate athlete's foot and nail fungus / helps skin to heal quicker and serves as a topical antibiotic when applied to cuts, wounds, and burns; may be added to distilled water and sprayed onto the area 2x a day for up to 5 days for this purpose / for Chronic Fatigue Syndrome and Epstein Barr virus, tea tree is best blended with peppermint essential oil and applied neat to the soles of the feet 2x daily for 1 week then stopping for five days before resuming; *this method and pattern of use seems to work best when employed every other month* / apply neat to the soles of the feet for nervous exhaustion from stress / apply neat to the soles of the feet combined with lavender to bring the body out of shock / a small amount applied with a cotton swab can be applied to warts / a few drops added to distilled water in a spray bottle makes an effective, healing facial spritzer and disinfectant for acne

Practical Uses: 3 drops added to water will help house plants fight fungus and molds and to recover from such / 30 drops added to distilled water and

borax will eliminate molds from surfaces / makes a highly effective house cleaner, especially when combined with peppermint or lavender / a drop or two added to warm water makes a highly effective mouthwash for gum troubles and to reduce plaque; can be combined with a drop of lemongrass or spearmint for a more pleasant scent and taste

Vibrational Influence: invites purity / deep cleans on the energetic level

Emotional Influence: calming to the nervous system and emotions

Synergistic to: white thyme, ravensara, clove, organic lemon, lemongrass, peppermint

Chakra Correspondence: root, solar plexus

Cosmetic Use: added to numerous soaps, cleansers, shampoos, lotions, First-Aid products, and skin preparations for its antimicrobial and healing action

Source and Parts Used: leaves from the tree

Tip: Tea tree oil's medicinal aroma can be tempered if diluted or combined with pleasant-smelling essential oils like lemon, lemongrass, and lavender. It can also be substituted with rosalina essential oil.

Thyme, White (Thymus vulgaris)

Scent: pungent and herbaceous

Clinical Uses: fungal, viral, and bacterial infections / tonsillitis / snoring / tonic for the nervous system / post-viral fatigue and weakness / food poisoning

Body Systems Affected: immune, nervous

Inhalation Effect: 1-2 drops added to a steam and inhaled is helpful for tonsillitis as well as sinus infections and pain Tip: use sparingly to avoid irritation

Dermal Effect: apply neat to the soles of the feet for all infectious diseases and tonsillitis; especially effective when combined with tea tree or lemon essential oil / apply neat to the soles of the feet to prevent or decrease

snoring; apply at bedtime / apply neat to the soles of the feet for systemic candida and overgrowth of yeast in the intestines / apply 2 drops neat to the soles of the feet for food poisoning; apply 2x daily

Practical Uses: highly effective household cleaner and air freshener / highly effective against Salmonella on surfaces

Vibrational Influence: clears the energy field of people and places

Emotional Influence: calming to the nerves

Synergistic to: tea tree, oregano, clove, lavender

Chakra Correspondence: root, solar plexus

Cosmetic Use: N/A

Source and Parts Used: leaves and stems of the aromatic plant

Caution: *White thyme essential oil is very potent and must be kept from mucus membranes **e.g.** eyes, nose, mouth, and genital area.*

Tsuga (Tsuga canadensis)

a.k.a. Canadian Hemlock, Spruce Hemlock and White Hemlock

Scent: deep evergreen, pine-like

Clinical Uses: pain reduction in cases of rheumatoid arthritis / muscle pain / urinary tract infections / lung support

Body Systems Affected: urinary, respiratory

Inhalation Effect: may be diffused into the air via nebulizer for respiratory conditions such as coughs, lung infections, cold, and flu

Dermal Effect: dilute well and apply to joints and muscles to reduce pain in cases of arthritic conditions, chronic pain syndromes, and strains / dilute well and apply to kidney area and low back for urinary tract infections; also apply neat to the soles of the feet

Practical Uses: household cleaner, air freshener, room spray, and added to potpourri

Vibrational Influence: holds the energy of protection and stability

Emotional Influence: dispels feelings of defeat and futility / encourages resilience and stamina in the face of adversity

Synergistic to: pine bark, pine needle, black spruce, sandalwood, frankincense

Chakra Correspondence: root, solar plexus

Cosmetic Use: used in perfumery

Source and Parts Used: needles (leaves) and twigs of the conifer tree

Caution: *Do not use tsuga essential oil on young children, for their skin may be too sensitive.*

Tip: Tsuga essential oil has received a negative reputation as being potentially toxic because it is too often confused with poison hemlock. Poison hemlock is a perennial meadow plant while tsuga is in the botanical family of Pinaceae (evergreen *trees*) and safe. Use properly diluted to avoid skin irritation.

Vanilla (Vanilla planifolia)

Scent: vanilla, sweet and warm with subtle smoky undertones

Clinical Uses: stimulation of the neurotransmitter serotonin / symptoms of mild-moderate depression / mood fluctuations associated with premenstrual syndrome / anxiety and excessive worry

Body Systems Affected: nervous

Inhalation Effect: lifts the mood and calms anxiety by increasing serotonin production almost immediately / excellent when used in an aroma locket / especially effective when combined with lavender and/or cacao

Dermal Effect: N/A

Practical Uses: N/A

Vibrational Influence: carries the energies of peace and contentment

Emotional Influence: soothes states of weepiness, frustration, and irritability / provides a sense of comfort, stability, and calm / relaxes the body and mind / inspires and improves sensual awareness

Synergistic to: lavender, cacao

Chakra Correspondence: heart

Cosmetic Use: used in perfumery

Source and Parts Used: from the pods of the orchid vine

Tip: *100% of fragrance oils marketed as "vanilla" are synthetic and possess zero therapeutic value. Look for solvent-extracted vanilla oleoresin/vanilla absolute, or finer quality, solvent-free vanilla CO2 for the true vanilla used in aromatherapy. Vanilla is available in diluted form and quite affordable, though the concentrated CO2 or absolute is worth the cost for its full aromatic benefits.*

Valerian (Valeriana Officinalis)

Scent: pungent, musty

Clinical Uses: moderate-severe anxiety / stubborn insomnia / rheumatoid arthritis / Parkinson's disease

Body Systems Affected: nervous/limbic

Inhalation Effect: for those who do not dislike the aroma of valerian, it can induce deep calm and emotional wellbeing / excellent to induce sleep and combat insomnia when inhaled before bed; combine with Atlas cedar or lavender for an enhanced effect needed for stubborn insomnia

Dermal Effect: provides deep and extraordinary relaxation when applied neat to the soles of the feet or diluted and used in massage / induces deep sleep when applied neat to the soles of the feet before bed / may be helpful for Parkinson's disease when applied neat to the soles of the feet or used in massage modalities / highly effective for panic attacks, severe anxiety, and traumatic emotional upset

Practical Uses: N/A

Vibrational Influence: resonates with the frequency of calm stability

Emotional Influence: brings deep peace and inner stillness / calms the physical symptoms of anxiety, panic, and emotional extremes

Synergistic to: spikenard, Atlas cedarwood, ylang ylang

Chakra Correspondence: solar plexus, heart

Cosmetic Use: can be used to further the healing of closed wounds and rashes

Source and Parts Used: from the rhizomes of the plant

Caution: *Do not use if taking pharmaceutical antidepressants and/or anti-anxiety medications. Do not apply to open wounds.*

Tip: Combining valerian essential oil with sweet ylang ylang makes the aroma of this oil more pleasant, and the combination is excellent to use with Swedish massage or applied neat for deep, sedative properties.

<u>Vetiver</u> (Vetiveria zizanoides)

Scent: deep and earthy similar to freshly-turned soil and roots

Clinical Uses: women's hormone balance of estrogen-progesterone for premenstrual syndrome, perimenopause, and menopause / connective tissue weakness / stimulation of red blood cell production / anxiety, especially related to the menstrual cycle / insomnia, especially hormone-related / fluctuating heart and breathing rate / anxiety or panic that leads to difficult breathing or hyperventilation

Body Systems Affected: hormonal, musculoskeletal, nervous

Inhalation Effect: brings equilibrium to the heart rate and slows breathing when needed / calms and balances the nervous system / calms excessive thoughts or worry / <u>Tip</u>: 1 drop on the palm of the hand and inhaled will regulate breathing and reset the body during severe anxiety or panic attacks

Dermal Effect: diluted and used in massage to balance the nervous system / diluted and used in massage to help improve collagen of the skin / applied neat to the soles of the feet to systemically improve connective tissue strength and integrity / may be helpful when applied neat to the soles of the feet or diluted and used in massage to calm the nerves, promote better sleep, and ease premenstrual syndrome / apply neat to balance estrogen and progesterone in the body / apply neat to the soles of the feet to support the blood and red blood cell production

Practical Uses: used in potpourri

Vibrational Influence: helps to integrate masculine and feminine energies within the human trinity of body-mind-spirit / provides a sense of certainty and security where there is instability

Emotional Influence: encourages self-worth, self-esteem, strong identity, and confidence / helps replenish energy reserves in cases of emotional exhaustion, especially if accompanied by nervousness or worry / calms the mind / minimizes the desperate need for perfection

Synergistic to: sandalwood, myrrh, clary sage, geranium, vitex, pine needle

Chakra Correspondence: root, navel/sacral, solar plexus, heart

Cosmetic Use: used as a fixative or base note in perfumery and some skin preparations

Source and Parts Used: roots of the grass

Vitex (Agnus castus)

a.k.a. Chaste Berry

Scent: woody with peppery overtones

Clinical Uses: polycystic ovarian syndrome / progesterone production for female hormone balance / uterine fibroids / luteal-phase defects of the female reproductive system that may lead to miscarriages and infertility / Parkinson's disease / stimulation of dopamine production / harmony of the endocrine system / hormone balance in men and women / estrogen

dominance / enlarged prostate (BPH) / men's hair loss / prostate cancer / regulation of the pituitary gland / Tourette syndrome

Body Systems Affected: reproductive, endocrine, nervous

Inhalation Effect: highly useful for reducing discomfort of menopause when inhaled multiple times a day / may stimulate the pituitary and pineal glands, especially when combined with sandalwood or frankincense / may stimulate dopamine and highly effective for reducing symptoms of Parkinson's disease when combined with dermal use of the essential oil; can be diffused via nebulizer for best results / may be helpful for Tourette syndrome

Dermal Effect: diluted and used in massage, brings harmony to the endocrine system including reproductive organs, thyroid, and adrenals / relieves premenstrual symptoms when applied neat to the soles of the feet / may be helpful in preventing miscarriages, decreasing fibroids, and balancing conditions of estrogen-dominance / stimulates dopamine and extremely helpful for reducing symptoms of Parkinson's disease when applied neat to the soles of the feet, diluted and applied along the spine, and used in conjunction with inhalation of the oil / may be useful in cases of enlarged prostate and prostate cancer in men / balances hormones of the male reproductive system / regulation of the pituitary gland / may be highly useful in balancing the female reproductive system to increase fertility / may be helpful for Tourette syndrome when applied neat to the soles of the feet

Practical Uses: N/A

Vibrational Influence: may promote clairvoyance due to its effect on the pituitary and pineal glands

Emotional Influence: N/A

Synergistic to: vetiver, geranium

Chakra Correspondence: root, navel/sacral, brow

Cosmetic Use: N/A

Source and Parts Used: berries of the tree also known as chaste tree and monk's pepper

Notes: Vitex essential oil has been shown to be more effective for hormone regulation and reducing symptoms of menopause without the serious health risks and side effects of pharmaceutical hormone replacement therapy (HRT). According to French physician Dr. Jean Claude LaPraz, vitex is capable of reducing symptoms of Parkinson's disease by 89%. According to some sources, vitex essential oil has been shown to decrease symptoms of Tourette syndrome.

<u>Wintergreen</u> (Gaultheria procumbens)

Scent: pungent, sweet menthol similar to root beer

Clinical Uses: osteoarthritis / muscle and joint pain / sinus pressure and pain/ sciatica

Body Systems Affected: musculoskeletal, respiratory, nervous

Inhalation Effect: stimulates mental alertness / improves the mood / <u>Caution</u>: *use in minute amounts and not habitually*

Dermal Effect: reduces arthritis, muscle, and joint pain when diluted and applied to the area; use minimally and not habitually / combine with eucalyptus for best and safest results / useful for sciatic pain when diluted and applied to the lower back, sacrum, and buttock

Practical Uses: excellent when small amounts are added to air fresheners and household cleaners

Vibrational Influence: clears the energy field of places and people / useful for clearing the energetic space of a room after a large gathering of people

Emotional Influence: lifts the mood and inspires optimism

Synergistic to: sweet birch, eucalyptus globulus

Chakra Correspondence: N/A

Cosmetic Use: N/A

Source and Parts Used: leaves of the aromatic shrub

Caution: *Wintergreen is equal to liquid aspirin. Individuals allergic or sensitive to aspirin should not use wintergreen essential oil. Individuals on blood thinners and those with epilepsy/seizure disorders should not use wintergreen essential oil. Do not use wintergreen on children. Wintergreen is often used and sold as birch essential oil. Both share very similar chemical compounds; these compounds can accumulate in the body and can be harmful if used consistently over time. To be on the safe side, use very sparingly and do not use these oils daily or habitually in dermal applications.*

Yarrow, Blue (Achillea millefolium)

Scent: deeply herbaceous with medicinal undertones

Clinical Uses: boils and wounds / irritated skin conditions / allergies and hay fever symptoms / liver support / gallbladder pain / effects of radiation therapy / adult stomachache and intestinal bloating

Body Systems Affected: dermal, nervous, endocrine, immune, gastro-intestinal

Inhalation Effect: soothes anger, grief, and loneliness

Dermal Effect: dilute and apply to the abdomen for stomachache and bloating in adults / dilute and apply to upper right abdomen for gallbladder pain / apply neat to the soles of the feet for allergy and hay fever symptoms; especially effective when combined with lavender / apply neat to the soles of the feet to support liver function // apply neat to the soles of the feet to ease menstrual discomfort / useful to ease the discomfort of radiation treatment / add to distilled water in a spray bottle to reduce inflammation, speed healing of the skin, and stop bleeding in early stages of healing; helpful for stubborn boils

Practical Uses: repels ticks

Vibrational Influence: highly protective / shields the auric field and creates a strong energetic barrier

Emotional Influence: brings equilibrium to the nervous system after intense, angry outbursts / comforts during times of grief / minimizes resentment

Synergistic to: lavender, German chamomile

Chakra Correspondence: root, solar plexus, heart, throat

Cosmetic Use: used in lotions, carrier oils, aloe vera, and distilled water (as a spray) to calm skin inflammation and to heal and rejuvenate skin cells

Source and Parts Used: flowering tops of the aromatic plant

Caution: *Individuals on blood thinners should avoid dermal use of yarrow essential oil.*

Tip: Blue yarrow is a beautiful, natural shade of blue.

Ylang Ylang (Cananga odorata)

Scent: sweet and heady, similar to jasmine without jasmine's subtle vanilla undertones

Clinical Uses: nervousness and anxiety / internal trembling / heart palpitations from overwrought nerves or hormonal swings in women / regulation of heart rhythm / insomnia / balancing adrenalin in the body / sexual response in women and men / dental pain

Body Systems Affected: nervous

Inhalation Effect: calms accelerated heart rate or breath / reduces panic attacks and anxiety / instantly stops internal trembling when inhaled simultaneously with neroli essential oil / balances the nervous system and helpful for hormonal states of anxiety, especially nocturnal physical anxiety / promotes sleep / enhances orgasmic response in women and men / calms the body after outbursts of temper

Dermal Effect: diluted and applied along the spine will reduce anxiety and reduce frequency of panic attacks / diluted and used in Swedish massage will calm the nervous system and balance excessive adrenalin and other stress hormones / applied neat to the soles of the feet will support the nervous system during times of stress or hormonal fluctuation / helps

reduce dental pain when diluted and rubbed along the jawline when applied prior to dental visits

Practical Uses: nice scent to use for clothes when sprinkled generously onto a damp wash cloth and added with wet clothes in the dryer

Vibrational Influence: invites high-frequency energies / resonates with the angelic kingdom

Emotional Influence: improves disposition / decreases irritability and desire for confrontation

Synergistic to: frankincense, Roman chamomile, jasmine, rosewood

Chakra Correspondence: navel/sacral, heart, crown

Cosmetic Use: used in perfumery / beneficial for oily and acne-prone skin

Source and Parts Used: flowers from the tropical tree

Tip: Also known as "poor man's jasmine," ylang ylang is one of the headiest floral essential oils. There are three distillations of the flowers, and the essential oils are sold as: <u>Ylang Ylang Extra</u> or Super = first pressing which yields the finest aroma and highest content of *linalool* that is responsible for the oil's calming effects, <u>Ylang Ylang 3rd Pressing</u> = the last pressing, considered inferior to Ylang Extra but still a potent and effective oil, and <u>Ylang Ylang Complete</u> = contains all pressings.

III

SYNERGISTIC DERMAL FORMULAS
FOR PHYSICAL WELLBEING

Boosting immunity. Hormone balance. Better sleep. Improved circulation. Pain & stress reduction. Chronic conditions. Fibromyalgia

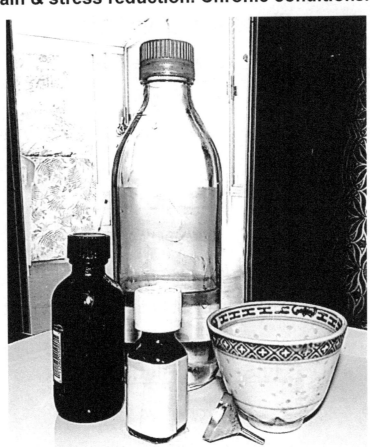

FLU and COLD SEASON IMMUNITY BOOSTERS

The following blends are designed to enhance immunity before and during the typical flu and cold season as well as reliable blends to improve immunity against other viruses. For best results, choose one to use daily for a week and then switch off so the body doesn't build up resistance to it. Essential oils are like armor, increasing the body's frequency, therefore, boosting immune response. These blends can also be used during illness but work best as a preventative measure.

Flu Season Blend #1:

2 drops organic lemon

1 drop clove

Apply neat to the soles of the feet before bed or any other time.

Flu Season Blend #2:

2 drops organic lemon

2 drops tea tree

Apply neat to the soles of the feet before bed or any other time.

Flu Season Blend #3:

1 drop clove

2 drops juniper berry

1 drop organic lemon

Apply neat to the soles of the feet before bed or any other time.

Flu Season Blend #4:

2 drops lavender

2 drops tea tree

2 drops organic lemon

Apply neat to the soles of the feet before bed or any other time.

Viral Defense Blend #1:

2 drops ravensara

2 drops tea tree

2 drops organic lemon

Apply neat to the soles of the feet. **Tip:** This blend is especially useful for chicken pox and shingles, both as prevention and management.

Viral Defense Blend #2:

2 drops ravensara

2 drops clove

2 drops geranium

Apply neat to the soles of the feet. **Tip:** This blend is especially useful for chicken pox and shingles, both as prevention and management.

General Immune Booster and Vitality Blend:

2 drops peppermint

2 drops organic lemon

Apply neat to the soles of the feet.

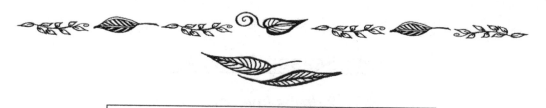

IMPROVING BLOOD CIRCULATION

Blood Circulation Blend #1:

3 drops peppermint

2 drops juniper berry

Apply neat to the soles of the feet in the morning, before traveling, or any other time. Excellent to use with massage modalities.

Blood Circulation Blend #2:

2 drops cypress

1 drop peppermint

Apply neat to the soles of the feet in the morning, before traveling, or any other time. **Tip:** This blend is especially good for individuals with tendencies toward varicose veins. Excellent to use with massage modalities.

Blood Circulation Blend #3:

1 drop ginger

1 drop juniper berry

1 drop nutmeg

Apply neat to the soles of the feet in the morning, before traveling, or any other time. **Tip:** This blend is especially good for individuals who suffer from the cold. Excellent to use with massage modalities.

IMPROVING LYMPHATIC CIRCULATION

Lymph Blend #1:

3 drops cypress

1 drop juniper berry

1 drop geranium

Apply neat to the soles of the feet and/or diluted and
used with Swedish massage or other massage modalities designed for
lymph drainage.

Lymph Blend #2:

2 drops geranium

2 drops grapefruit

1 drop lemon

Apply neat to the soles of the feet.

Lymph Blend #3:

2 drops cypress

2 drops peppermint

1 drop celery seed

Apply neat to the soles of the feet and/or diluted and
used with Swedish massage or other massage modalities designed for
lymph drainage.

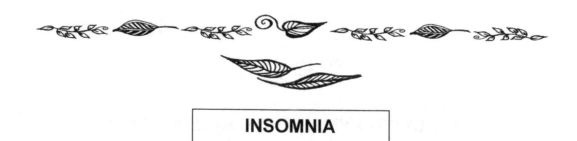

INSOMNIA

Insomnia Blend #1:

2 drops rosewood

1 drop lavender

1 drop ylang ylang

1 drop Atlas cedarwood

1 drop vetiver

Apply neat to the soles of the feet for best results. This can also be diluted in 1 teaspoon of carrier oil or lotion and applied along the spine. Apply 20 minutes before bed. Use consistently every evening. **Tip:** For best results, use relaxing essential oils via inhalation at intervals during the day. Lavender, frankincense, and neroli are good choices to use on a tissue or in an aroma locket for this purpose.

Insomnia Blend #2:

2 drops rosewood

2 drops Atlas cedarwood

2 drops spikenard

added to 1 teaspoon of carrier oil or lotion

Apply neat to the soles of the feet for best results. This can also be diluted in 1 teaspoon of carrier oil or lotion and applied along the spine. Apply 20 minutes before bed. Use consistently every evening. **Tip:** For best results, use relaxing essential oils via inhalation at intervals during the day. Lavender, frankincense, and neroli are good choices to use on a tissue or in an aroma locket for this purpose.

Insomnia Blend #3:

2 drops balsam fir

2 drops Atlas cedarwood

2 drops spikenard

1 drop rosewood (optional but recommended)

added to 1 teaspoon of carrier oil or lotion

Apply neat to the soles of the feet for best results. This can also be diluted in 1 teaspoon of carrier oil or lotion and applied along the spine. Apply 20 minutes before bed. Use consistently every evening. **Tip:** For best results, use relaxing essential oils via inhalation at intervals during the day. Lavender, frankincense, and neroli are good choices to use on a tissue or in an aroma locket for this purpose.

FEMALE WELLBEING- PMS

PMS Blend #1:

2 drops frankincense

2 drops geranium

2 drops clary sage

Apply neat to the soles of the feet and diluted along the spine and adrenal/kidney area during the week before menstruation. Highly effective for water retention, belly woes from hormonal shifts, and irritability.

PMS Blend #2:

2 drops cypress

2 drops clary sage

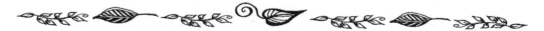

1 drop spearmint

Apply neat to the soles of the feet for a week before menstruation. Effective for water retention and moodiness.

PMS Blend #3:

2 drops bergamot

2 drops frankincense

1 drop geranium

Apply neat to the soles of the feet daily and inhale on a tissue or in an aroma locket for a week before menstruation. Effective for feelings of sadness and physical discomfort.

PMS Blend #4:

1 drop angelica root

1 drop geranium

1 drop lavender

Apply neat to the soles of the feet for a week before menstruation. Promotes a balancing effect.

FEMALE WELLBEING- PERIMENOPAUSE and MENOPAUSE

Women's Transition Blend #1:

2 drops geranium

2 drops clary sage

1 drop vitex

1 drop lavender

Apply neat to the soles of the feet during hormonal shifts, hot or cold flashes, digestive upset, and irritability. Promotes a balancing effect.

Women's Transition Blend #2:

1 drop geranium

1 drop clary sage

1 drop spearmint

Apply neat to the soles of the feet during hormonal shifts, hot or cold flashes, digestive upset, and irritability. Promotes a balancing effect.

Women's Transition Blend #3:

2 drops peppermint

2 drops clary sage

Apply neat to the soles of the feet to ease intensity of hot flashes. Promotes a balancing effect.

BREAST SUPPORT

Breast Support Blend #1:

1 drop lavender

1 drop frankincense

1 drop organic lemon

Dilute in 1 teaspoon *organic carrier oil* and rub into breasts daily.

Breast Support Blend #2:

2 drops frankincense

2 drops organic lemon

Dilute in 1 teaspoon *organic carrier oil* and rub into breasts daily.

COPING WITH STRESS

Morning Stress Blend #1:

2 drops black spruce

1 drop juniper berry

1 drop basil

Apply neat to the soles of the feet in the mornings.

Morning Stress Blend #2:

2 drops pine bark

1 drop patchouli

1 drop balsam fir

Apply neat to the soles of the feet in the mornings.

Evening Stress Blend #1:

2 drops lavender

2 drops balsam fir

Apply neat to the soles of the feet at bedtime.

Evening Stress Blend #2:

2 drops Roman chamomile

2 drops ylang ylang

1 drop geranium

Apply neat to the soles of the feet at bedtime.

MANAGING PAIN

Muscle Pain Blend #1:

3 drops peppermint

2 drops balsam fir

1 drop ginger

Dilute in 1 teaspoon of carrier oil or lotion and apply to affected area up to 4x a day with a few hours between applications. **Tip:** Omit ginger essential oil if it is contraindicated; this blend will still be highly effective.

Muscle Pain Blend #2:

3 drops juniper berry

2 drops balsam fir

2 drops eucalyptus globulus

Dilute in 1 teaspoon of carrier oil or lotion and apply to affected area up to 4x a day with a few hours between applications.

Muscle Pain Blend #3:

3 drops spearmint

2 drops pine needle

2 drops lavender

Dilute in 1 teaspoon of carrier oil or lotion and apply to affected area up to 4x a day with a few hours between applications.

Muscle Pain Blend #4:

3 drops ginger

2 drops spearmint

1 drop lemongrass

Dilute in 1 teaspoon of carrier oil or lotion and apply to affected area up to 4x a day with a few hours between applications.

Osteoarthritis Pain Blend #1:

3 drops eucalyptus globulus

2 drops balsam fir

2 drops peppermint

1 drop lavender

Dilute in 1 teaspoon of carrier oil or lotion and apply to affected area up to 3x a day with a few hours between applications.

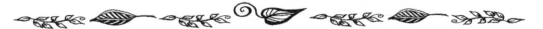

Osteoarthritis Pain Blend #2:

4 drops copaiba

2 drops frankincense

2 drops balsam fir

Dilute in 1 teaspoon of carrier oil or lotion and apply to affected area up to 4x a day with a few hours between applications.

.

Osteoarthritis Pain Blend #3:

3 drops juniper berry

2 drops lemon eucalyptus

*1 drop sweet birch or wintergreen

Dilute in 1 teaspoon of carrier oil or lotion and apply to affected area up to 2x a day with a few hours between applications. **Do not use more than 3 times a week due to the aspirin-like properties of sweet birch or wintergreen essential oil. Sweet birch and wintergreen can be substituted with balsam fir, spearmint, or pine needle.*

Rheumatoid Arthritis Pain Blend #1:

3 drops peppermint

3 drops sweet marjoram

2 drops Roman chamomile

Dilute in 1 teaspoon of carrier oil or lotion and apply to affected area up to 3x a day with a few hours between applications.

Rheumatoid Arthritis Pain Blend #2:

4 drops copaiba

4 drops helichrysum

Dilute in 1 teaspoon of carrier oil or lotion and apply to affected area up to 3x a day with a few hours between applications.

Rheumatoid Arthritis Pain Blend #3:

4 drops balsam fir

2 drops tsuga

1 drop bay laurel

Dilute in 1 teaspoon of carrier oil or lotion and apply to affected area up to 3x a day with a few hours between applications.

Post-Workout Soreness Blend #1:

4 drops balsam fir

3 drops spearmint

Dilute in 1 teaspoon of carrier oil or lotion and apply to affected area up to 2x a day with a few hours between applications. **Tip:** This blend is especially effective when used in sports massage. It can also be applied *before* working out or exercising to reduce soreness.

Post-Workout Soreness Blend #2:

2 drops balsam fir

3 drops spearmint

1 drop juniper berry

Dilute in 1 teaspoon of carrier oil or lotion and apply to affected area up to 2x a day with a few hours between applications. **Tip:** This blend is especially effective when used in sports massage. It can also be applied *before* working out or exercising to reduce soreness.

Tension Headache Blend #1:

1 drop lavender

1 drop spearmint

1 drop Roman chamomile

Dilute in a little carrier oil or lotion and apply to back of the neck, shoulders, and temples (avoiding the eyes) up to 3x a day with a few hours between applications.

Tension Headache Blend #2:

1 drop balsam fir

1 drop peppermint

1 drop basil

Dilute in a little carrier oil or lotion and apply to back of the neck, shoulders, and temples (avoiding the eyes) up to 3x a day with a few hours between applications.

Migraine Headache Blend #1:

2 drops rosewood

1 drop German chamomile

Apply neat to the soles of the feet and dilute in a little carrier oil or lotion and apply to back of the neck, shoulders, and temples up to 3x a day with a few hours between applications, provided the aromas are tolerated. Tip: For best results, apply this blend at the first indication of a migraine coming on. As a possible preventative, use this blend regularly 2x a week and alternate with other recommended blends.

Migraine Headache Blend #2:

1 drop basil

1 drop peppermint

1 drop helichrysum

Apply neat to the soles of the feet and dilute in a little carrier oil or lotion and apply to back of the neck, shoulders, and temples up to 3x a day with a few hours between applications, provided the aromas are tolerated. <u>Tip</u>: For best results, apply this blend at the first indication of a migraine coming on. As a possible preventative, use this blend regularly 2x a week and alternate with other recommended blends.

Fibromyalgia/Myofascial Pain Blend #1:

2 drops spearmint

2 drops balsam fir

1-2 drops ginger

1 drop juniper berry

Dilute in 1-2 teaspoons of carrier oil or lotion and apply to affected areas or all over the body 2x a day with a few hours between applications. Especially effective when used in massage modalities.

Fibromyalgia/Myofascial Pain Blend #2:

3 drops peppermint

2 drops balsam fir

2 drops pine needle

Dilute in 1-2 teaspoons of carrier oil or lotion and apply to affected areas or all over the body 2-3x a day with a few hours between applications. Especially effective when used in massage modalities.

Fibromyalgia/Myofascial Pain Blend #3:

2 drops ginger

3 drops black spruce

Dilute in 1-2 teaspoons of carrier oil or lotion and apply to affected areas or all over the body 2x a day with a few hours between applications. Especially effective when used in massage modalities.

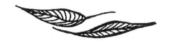

COPING WITH SEASONAL ALLERGIES

Seasonal Allergy Blend #1:

2 drops lavender

2 drops lemon

1 drop juniper

Apply neat to the soles of the feet every morning and to the palms of the hands whenever needed (for the palms, use 1 drop of each essential oil.) **Tip:** Also very useful for food sensitivities.

Seasonal Allergy Blend #2:

2 drops lavender

2 drops eucalyptus

1 drop peppermint

Apply neat to the soles of the feet every morning and to the palms of the

hands whenever needed (for the palms, use 1 drop of each essential oil.) Especially effective when used in Swedish massage. <u>Tip</u>: This blend is also effective for mold and dust sensitivity.

FOOD SENSITIVITIES

Food Sensitivity Blend:

1 drop lavender

1 drop lemon

1 drop peppermint

Apply neat to the soles of the feet every morning and to the palms of the hands whenever needed. <u>Tip</u>: This blend is highly useful for dairy and wheat sensitivity. Used before and after consumption to ease reactive symptoms.

MOLD and CHEMICAL SENSITIVITY

Sensitivity Blend:

2 drops lemon eucalyptus

2 drops peppermint

Inhale and apply neat to the soles of the feet every morning and to the palms of the hands as soon as possible after exposure. (For the palms, use 1 drop of each essential oil).

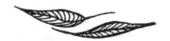

CHOLESTEROL BALANCE

Cholesterol Blend #1:

3 drops organic grapefruit

2 drops clary sage

1 drop lemon

Apply neat to the soles of the feet daily.

Cholesterol Blend #2:

3 drops myrrh

3 drops carrot seed

Apply neat to the soles of the feet daily.

High Blood Pressure Blend #1:

3 drops lemon

3 drops lavender

Apply neat to the soles of the feet daily.

High Blood Pressure Blend #2:

2 drops ginger

2 drops lemon

Apply neat to the soles of the feet daily.

High Blood Pressure Blend #3:

3 drops may chang

3 drops lavender

2 drops melissa

Apply neat to the soles of the feet daily.

High Blood Pressure Blend #4:

2 drops sweet marjoram

3 drops davana

2 drops lavender

Apply neat to the soles of the feet daily.

Low Blood Pressure Blend #1:

2 drops peppermint

2 drop hyssop

1 drop lavender

Apply neat to the soles of the feet daily.

Low Blood Pressure Blend #2:

2 drops peppermint

1 drop eucalyptus

Apply neat to the soles of the feet daily.

DIGESTIVE EASE

Indigestion Blend:

4 drops peppermint

2 drops lavender

diluted in a teaspoon or more of carrier oil and applied to abdomen.

Tip: Good for bellyaches, distention/bloating, intestinal rumbling.

Use half the recommended number of essential oils for older children;

substitute peppermint with spearmint in half dosage and double dilution for younger children.

Intestinal Blend:

3 drops peppermint

1 drops sweet orange or tangerine

1 drop patchouli

1 drop clove

diluted in a teaspoon or more of carrier oil and applied to abdomen up to 3x a day. **Tip:** good for intestinal rumbling, diarrhea, and discomfort from constipation. Use half the recommended number of essential oils for older children; substitute peppermint with spearmint in half dosage and double dilution for younger children.

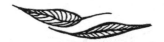

MEMORY BOOSTERS and STUDY AIDS

Memory Booster Blend #1:

1 drop peppermint

1 drop rosemary

1 drop spearmint

Inhale at 5 minute intervals throughout the day to boost memory, while studying, or before taking exams. The essential oils can be applied to a tissue, the palms of the hands, or used in an aroma locket.

Memory Booster Blend #2:

1 drop basil

1 drop spearmint

Inhale for 5 minute intervals throughout the day to boost memory, while studying, or before taking exams. The essential oils can be applied to a tissue, the palms of the hands, or used in an aroma locket.

Memory Booster Blend #3:

1 drop grapefruit

1 drop neroli

Inhale at intervals throughout the day to boost memory, while studying, or before taking exams. The essential oils can be applied to a tissue, the palms of the hands, or used in an aroma locket.

Memory Booster Blend #4:

1 drop clove

1 drop nutmeg

Inhale at brief intervals throughout the day to boost memory, while studying, or before taking exams. The essential oils can be applied to a tissue, the palms of the hands, or used in an aroma locket.

Memory Booster Blend #5:

1 drop cacao

1 drop coffee bean

Inhale at brief intervals throughout the day to boost memory, while studying, or before taking exams. The essential oils can be applied to a tissue, the palms of the hands, or used in an aroma locket.

MORNING & EVENING COMBINATIONS for
CHRONIC FATIGUE SYNDROME /
MYALGIC ENCEPHALOMYELITIS

The following blends support individuals coping with CFIDS/ME. For best results, it is recommended to rotate the blends. **e.g.** use one combo for 4 days and then switch to another.

Essential Oil Duo 1

CFIDS/ME Morning Blend:

3 drops peppermint

3 drops tea tree

Apply neat to the soles of the feet in the morning.

CFIDS/ME Evening Blend:

3 drops frankincense

3 drops lavender

2 drops rosewood

Apply neat to the soles of the feet in the evening before bed. **Tip:** This blend is especially supportive of the nervous and endocrine systems.

Essential Oil Duo 2

CFIDS/ME Morning Blend:

2 drops rosewood

2 drops tea tree

1 drop geranium

Apply neat to the soles of the feet in the morning.

CFIDS/ME Evening Blend:

2 drops rosewood

2 drops balsam fir

1 drop geranium

1 drop frankincense

Apply neat to the soles of the feet in the evenings before bed.

Tip: This blend is especially supportive of the endocrine and immune systems.

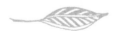

CHRONIC FATIGUE SYNDROME/MYALGIC ENCEPHALOMYELITIS DAILY BLEND

The following blend is a simpler approach to support individuals coping with CFIDS/ME. For best results, apply neat to the soles of the feet 2x daily for 1 week then stop for five days before resuming; *this method and pattern of use seems to work best when employed every other month.*

CFIDS/ME Daily Blend:

2 drops peppermint

2 drops tea tree

Apply neat to the soles of the feet in the morning and evening.

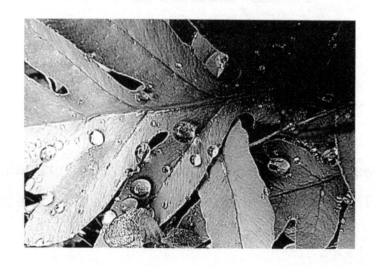

IV

SYNERGISTIC
DERMAL & INHALATION FORMULAS
FOR EMOTIONAL WELLBEING

**Anxiety. Panic attacks. Symptoms of depression. Grief/transition.
Healing the past. Self-worth issues. Emotional stress. Cravings**

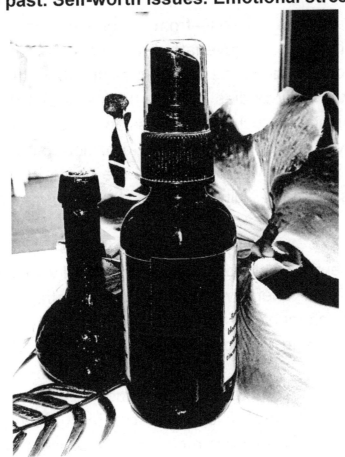

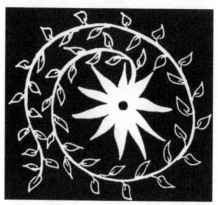

Chemical Messengers and Emotional Equilibrium

Our bodies never get a day off—from second to second, their complex functions fight off disease, rejuvenate, break down, process, and maintain all the workings of survival. Understanding a little about the nervous system can help us to know our bodies and the origins of emotional and psycho-physiological conditions such as depression, chronic anxiety and panic attacks, obsessive compulsive and eating disorders, and mood fluctuation. It can also help us to know how to fortify the nervous system to possibly help our brains be less vulnerable to devastating diseases such as Alzheimer's.

A section on essential oil blends and our emotional wellbeing would not be as useful without a brief overview about neurotransmitters—chemical messengers that communicate with nerve cells and play a vital and intricate role in both physical and emotional wellbeing.

There are numerous neurotransmitters, and they come in two kinds—*inhibitory* and *excitatory*. Too little or too much of any given neurotransmitter can foster poor memory and concentration, depression, high-risk behavior, carbohydrate and sugar cravings, anxiety and panic attacks, insomnia, mood changes, seasonal affective disorder (S.A.D.), ADHD, irritability, predisposition toward addiction, and so much more. Some of these neurotransmitters are serotonin, dopamine, acetylcholine,

norepinephrine, and GABA. **Serotonin**—an *inhibitory* neurotransmitter—plays a major role in taming excessive production of excitatory chemicals that are responsible for low immunity, disrupted sleep cycles, sugar cravings, and heightened pain. Regular consumption of coffee and other stimulants, prolonged stress, hormonal changes, and poor diet compromise and deplete our serotonin levels. In the simplest terms, serotonin imbalance directly affects many functions in the body including digestion as well as emotional wellbeing; when it is disrupted, it can be evident in many ways ranging from hormonal moodiness to eating disorders such as bulimia. **Dopamine,** both inhibitory and excitatory (and also a hormone) keeps memory sharp and makes us feel alert and motivated. Caffeine, alcohol, and some recreational drugs jumpstart dopamine briefly, but habitual consumption or use further depletes dopamine until it takes more and more of the substance to feel any effect. This is why dopamine and other neurotransmitters play a critical role in addiction and addictive behaviors. **GABA** is the body's natural, magical substance of sedation and should kick in when another neurotransmitter such as norepinephrine keeps firing off causing severe anxiety or insomnia.

Playing a leading role in this physiological production is the *amygdala,* a portion of the brain that helps us to feel fear so we know when we are in danger. The amygdala is responsible for associating sights, smells, sounds, tastes and sensation with unpleasant memories and/or trauma. When stimulated by certain smells, sounds, or other recognized stimuli, the amygdala sends out chemical messengers to trigger the body into the fight or flight stress response. Healthy amygdalas know when to turn off after danger passes, but if stress is traumatic and/or prolonged, the amygdala accumulates more and more associations in the memory bank, and this survival mechanism gets stuck on overdrive. Over time, in certain individuals, the amygdala perceives more and more stimuli as threatening and reacts accordingly. The adrenals, our stress glands, do what they are told via neurotransmitters and pump out adrenaline and cortisol. The result can be chronic anxiety with or without panic attacks, post-traumatic stress disorder (PTSD), and according to some theories, exhaustion and

syndromes such as Chronic Fatigue Immune Dysfunction (also known as Myalgic Encephalomyelitis.)

The more we can show the amygdala that it is "okay" to shut off these responses when they are not needed, the more our bodies can finally rest, sleep deeply, digest properly, and shift our emotions to more positive states. This is where essential oils can be highly beneficial and in some cases, life-changing.

The body is always in flux, and this is why certain essential oils work better for us at different times. Life is stressful, and certain circumstances and triggers do not always affect us the same way. Sometimes we get headaches or anxiety, nightmares or irritability, obsessive thoughts or indescribable sadness; life is changing, and we are changing beings. A single essential oil that helped us last week or last year may not help us today. This is where synergy comes into play and offers the most latitude for healing to take place. Synergistic blends consist of essential oils that work in harmony with each other, therefore creating a more powerful and direct end result. For example, if a woman experiences heightened anxiety during ovulation or just prior to menstruation, an essential oil that helps to balance hormones can be added to a synergistic blend for anxiety. Or if intense cravings for sweets or carbohydrates accompany sadness, an essential oil known to boost serotonin can be added to a synergistic blend for melancholy.

Both dermal and inhalation applications have a profound effect on the nervous system, inhalation being the most immediate. As a rule of thumb, inhalation is recommended for any acute state such as a panic attack or stage fright associated with public speaking, while dermal blends are recommended as fortification and maintenance between extremes. Both methods work even better when used compatibly. Everyone has specific, individual needs and chemistry, and it may take a little experimenting to see what works best as well as knowing how much of a particular essential oil should be added to a blend. Practice, study, experimentation, and taking note of the body's responses are all important.

The following recommended blends are based on synergy—essential oils working together as a whole. Emotional issues need time to surface, to heal, and to integrate the past with the present. When using essential oils for emotional wellbeing, they must be used consistently for best results. Symptoms of anxiety, transitions such as grief, and cravings respond more quickly with aromatherapy—sometimes within seconds, minutes, or hours but are also recommended to be applied with consistency.

BLENDS FOR ACUTE GRIEF

The use of essential oils for acute grief can never lessen or numb the emotional pain of deep loss, but it can help our physical bodies weather the storm much better by nourishing neurotransmitter production. Emotionally, essential oils comfort, lift our frequency, and envelop us in comfort when we need it most.

Grief Blend #1:

2 drops sandalwood

2 drops rosewood

1 drop geranium

added to 1 teaspoon of carrier oil or lotion

This can be applied along the spine, the sacrum (at the base of the spine), and the heart center (area of the sternum between the breasts). Apply morning and evening or with massage modalities. The same combination can be applied to the palms of the hands and inhaled OR *undiluted* when added to a tissue or aroma locket using: 1 *drop sandalwood, 1 drop rosewood, and 1 drop geranium. Inhale as needed.* ***Tip:** *Sandalwood*

essential oil is available in diluted form at a fraction of the cost and is suitable for blends such as this.

Grief Blend #2:

1 drop cypress

2 drops myrrh

1 drop frankincense

1 drop ylang ylang

added to 1 teaspoon of carrier oil or lotion

This can be applied along the spine, the sacrum (at the base of the spine), and the heart center (area of the sternum between the breasts). The same combination can be applied to the palms of the hands and inhaled OR *undiluted* when added to a tissue or aroma locket using: 1 *drop cypress, 1 drop myrrh, and 1 drop frankincense, and 1 drop geranium*

Tip: *Myrrh essential oil is available in diluted form at a fraction of the cost and is suitable for blends such as this.*

Grief Blend #3:

2 drops ylang ylang

1 drop lavender

1 drop geranium

added to 1 teaspoon of carrier oil or lotion

This can be applied along the spine, the sacrum (at the base of the spine), and the heart center (area of the sternum between the breasts). The same combination can be applied to the palms of the hands and inhaled OR *undiluted* when added to a tissue or aroma locket using: 1 *drop ylang ylang, 1 drop lavender, and 1 drop geranium*

Tip: *This blend is especially suitable for cases of shock.*

BLENDS FOR SEPARATION, BREAK-UPS, & DEEP DISAPPOINTMENT

Essential oils can help us over rough waters of the heart and keep our serotonin and dopamine levels more plentiful. It is a fact that when we are in love or infatuated, our dopamine levels are at an all-time high flooding our system with chemicals that are considered to be the body's natural opiates. When a relationship ends, our feel-good neurotransmitters drop considerably and we are in some ways, subject to withdrawal from *our own chemicals*. The following blends can ensure an easier passage physiologically and emotionally.

Heartache Blend #1:

3 drops rose otto or absolute

2 drops vanilla absolute

1 drop lavender

added to 1 teaspoon of carrier oil or lotion

This can be applied along the spine, the sacrum (at the base of the spine), and the heart center (area of the sternum between the breasts). The same combination can be applied to the palms of the hands and inhaled OR *undiluted* when added to a tissue or aroma locket using: 1 *drop lavender, 2 drops vanilla, and 1 drop rose*

Tip: *Rose essential oil is available in diluted form at a fraction of the cost and is suitable for blends such as this.*

Heartache Blend #2:

2 drops cacao essential oil

2 drops rose otto or absolute

1 drop ylang ylang

1 drop benzoin

added to 1 teaspoon of carrier oil or lotion

This can be applied along the spine, the sacrum (at the base of the spine), and the heart center (area of the sternum between the breasts). The same combination can be applied to the palms of the hands and inhaled OR *undiluted* when added to a tissue or aroma locket using: 1 *drop cacao, 1 drop rose, 1 drop ylang ylang, and 1 drop benzoin*

Tip: *Rose essential oil is available in diluted form at a fraction of the cost and is suitable for blends such as this. This blend is especially suitable for women and teens*

Heartache Blend #3:

2 drops Roman chamomile

1 drop lavender

1 drop sweet marjoram

added to 1 teaspoon of carrier oil or lotion

This can be applied along the spine, the sacrum (at the base of the spine), and the heart center (area of the sternum between the breasts). The same combination can be applied to the palms of the hands and inhaled OR *undiluted* when added to a tissue or aroma locket using: 1 *drop Roman chamomile, 1 drop lavender and 1 drop sweet marjoram*

Tip: *Roman chamomile essential oil is available in diluted form at a fraction of the cost and is suitable for blends such as this.*

GENERAL or MILD ANXIETY AND NERVOUSNESS

Anxiety Blend #1:

2 drops lavender

2 drops sweet orange

1 drop Roman chamomile

added to 1 teaspoon of carrier oil or lotion

This can be applied along the spine, the sacrum (at the base of the spine), and the solar plexus (upper abdomen.) The same combination can be applied to the palms of the hands and inhaled OR *undiluted* when added to a tissue or aroma locket using: *1 drop lavender, 1 drop sweet orange, and 1 drop Roman chamomile*

Tip: *Roman chamomile essential oil is available in diluted form at a fraction of the cost and is suitable for blends such as this.*

Anxiety Blend #2:

2 drops frankincense

1 drop vetiver

1 drop ylang ylang

added to 1 teaspoon of carrier oil or lotion

This can be applied along the spine, the sacrum (at the base of the spine), and the solar plexus (upper abdomen.) The same combination can be applied to the palms of the hands and inhaled OR *undiluted* when added to a tissue or aroma locket using: *1 drop frankincense, 1 drop vetiver, and 1 drop ylang ylang*

Anxiety Blend #3:

(good for stage fright, public speaking, or job interviews)

1 drop basil

1 drop lavender

1 drop sweet orange or tangerine

added to 1 teaspoon of carrier oil or lotion

This can be applied along the spine, the sacrum (at the base of the spine), and the solar plexus (upper abdomen.) The same combination can be applied to the palms of the hands and inhaled OR *undiluted* when added to a tissue or aroma locket using: *1 drop basil, 1 drop lavender, and 1 drop sweet orange or tangerine*

Anxiety Blend #4:

(for nervousness associated with the female menstrual cycle)
***for moderate-to-severe anxiety during hormonal times, see the next section*

3 drops rose absolute

2 drops neroli

1 drop geranium

added to 1 teaspoon of carrier oil or lotion

This can be applied along the spine, the sacrum (at the base of the spine), and the solar plexus (upper abdomen.) The same combination can be applied to the palms of the hands and inhaled OR *undiluted* when added to a tissue or aroma locket using: *2 drops rose, 1 drop neroli, and 1 drop geranium.*

Tip: *Both rose and neroli essential oils are available in diluted form at a fraction of the cost and are suitable for blends such as this.*

Panic Blend #1:

3 drops frankincense

2 drops ylang ylang

2 drops lavender

added to 1 teaspoon of carrier oil or lotion

This can be applied along the spine, the sacrum (at the base of the spine), and the solar plexus (upper abdomen.) Apply 2x a day, morning and evening or when needed. Apply neat to the soles of the feet for acute anxiety. The same combination can be applied to the palms of the hands and inhaled OR *undiluted* when added to a tissue or aroma locket using: 1 *drop frankincense, 1 drop ylang ylang, and 1 drop lavender*

Panic Blend #2:

2 drops Atlas cedarwood

2 drops spikenard

2 drops ylang ylang

1 drop frankincense

1 drop lavender

added to 1 teaspoon of carrier oil or lotion

This can be applied along the spine, the sacrum (at the base of the spine), and the solar plexus (upper abdomen.) Apply 2x a day, morning and evening or when needed. Apply neat to the soles of the feet for acute anxiety. The same combination can be applied to the palms of the hands and inhaled OR *undiluted* when added to a tissue or aroma locket: 1 *drop frankincense, 1 drop Atlas cedarwood, 1 drop lavender, 1 drop spikenard, and 1 drop ylang ylang*

Notes for massage therapists: *This blend is ideal for those suffering from panic and anxiety disorders. This blend often works when all else has failed to help ease symptoms. It is best applied from the cervical area to the coccyx, worked in gently along the spine and in the lamina grooves. For optimum results, this blend works best during a 90 minute massage with employed breathwork.*

Panic Blend #3:

3 drops ylang ylang

2 drops lavender

2 drops vetiver

added to 1 teaspoon of carrier oil or lotion

This can be applied along the spine, the sacrum (at the base of the spine), and the solar plexus (upper abdomen.) Apply 2x a day, morning and evening or when needed. Apply neat to the soles of the feet for acute anxiety. The same combination can be applied to the palms of the hands and inhaled OR *undiluted* when added to a tissue or aroma locket using: *1 drop ylang ylang, 1 drop lavender, 1 drop vetiver* **Tip:** This blend is especially useful for rapid heartbeat associated with moderate-severe anxiety.

Panic Blend #4:

(for intense anxiety associated with the female menstrual cycle, perimenopause, or menopause)

3 drops neroli

1 drop ylang ylang

1 drop geranium

1 drop frankincense

1 drop vetiver

added to 1 teaspoon of carrier oil or lotion

This can be applied along the spine, the sacrum (at the base of the spine), and the solar plexus (upper abdomen.) Apply neat to the soles of the feet for acute anxiety. The same combination can be applied to the palms of the hands and inhaled OR *undiluted* when added to a tissue or aroma locket using: *1 drop neroli, 1 drop ylang ylang, 1 drop geranium, 1 drop frankincense, and 1 drop vetiver*

Panic Blend #5:

(for intense anxiety associated with the female menstrual cycle, perimenopause, or menopause)

3 drops neroli

2 drops Atlas cedarwood

2 drops vetiver

added to 1 teaspoon of carrier oil or lotion

This can be applied along the spine, the sacrum (at the base of the spine), and the solar plexus (upper abdomen.) Apply neat to the soles of the feet for acute anxiety. The same combination can be applied to the palms of the hands and inhaled OR *undiluted* when added to a tissue or aroma locket using: *1 drop neroli, 1 drop Atlas cedarwood, and 1 drop vetiver*

SUGAR AND CARBOHYDRATE CRAVINGS

Cravings Blend #1:

1 drop cacao

1 drop lavender

233

1 drop rose absolute

Inhale whenever cravings surface and at intervals throughout the day. Can be used in the palm of the hands, on a tissue, or in an aroma locket for this purpose. **Tip:** This combination works well for chocolate cravings and cravings that accompany sadness or loneliness. Also good inhalation blend for hormonal cravings.

Cravings Blend #2:

1 drop grapefruit

1 drop lavender

1 drop sweet orange

Inhale whenever cravings surface and at intervals throughout the day. Can be used in the palm of the hands, on a tissue, or in an aroma locket for this purpose. **Tip:** This blend works especially well for sugar cravings.

Cravings Blend #3:

1 drop basil

1 drop lavender

1 drop clary sage

Inhale whenever cravings surface and at intervals throughout the day. Can be used in the palm of the hands, on a tissue, or in an aroma locket for this purpose. **Tip:** This blend works especially well for cravings that accompany apathy and low energy (e.g. afternoon slumps).

Cravings Blend #4:

2 drops cacao

1 drop ginger

Inhale whenever cravings surface and at intervals throughout the day. Can be used in the palm of the hands, on a tissue, or in an aroma locket for this purpose. **Tip:** This blend works especially well for cravings that accompany

apathy and low energy (e.g. rainy days, long winter days, and afternoon slumps.)

"The Blues": MELANCHOLY, APATHY, AND HOPELESSNESS

The Blues- Blend #1:

1 drop lavender

1 drop Roman chamomile

1 drop bergamot

Inhale at 5-10 minute intervals throughout the day. Can be used in the palm of the hands, on a tissue, or in an aroma locket for this purpose.

The Blues- Blend #2:

1 drop balsam fir

1 drop clove

1 drop sweet orange

Inhale at 5-10 minute intervals throughout the day. Can be used in the palm of the hands, on a tissue, or in an aroma locket for this purpose.

The Blues- Blend #3:

1 drop grapefruit

1 drop bergamot

1 drop ylang ylang

Inhale at 5-10 minute intervals throughout the day. Can be used in the palm of the hands, on a tissue, or in an aroma locket for this purpose.

The Blues- Blend #4:

1 drop sweet orange

1 drop lemon

1 drop lemongrass

Inhale at 5-10 minute intervals throughout the day. Can be used in the palm of the hands, on a tissue, or in an aroma locket for this purpose.

The Blues- Blend #5:

1 drop angelica

1 drop vetiver

1 drop ginger

Inhale at 5-10 minute intervals throughout the day. Can be used in the palm of the hands, on a tissue, or in an aroma locket for this purpose.

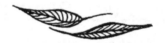

STABILITY DURING CHANGE

Stability Blend #1:

2 drops cypress

2 drops Atlas cedarwood

1 drop vetiver

Apply neat to the soles of the feet and/or dilute in 1 teaspoon of carrier oil or lotion and apply to the adrenal/kidney area and the sacrum. Can be used daily.

Stability Blend #2:

1 drop patchouli

1 drop frankincense

1 drop balsam fir

Apply neat to the soles of the feet and/or dilute in 1 teaspoon of carrier oil or lotion and apply to the adrenal/kidney area and the sacrum.
Can be used daily.

Coping with Trauma- Blend #1:

2 drops helichrysum

1 drop Roman chamomile

1 drop lavender

1 drop frankincense

Inhale at 5-10 minute intervals throughout the day. Can be used in the palm of the hands, on a tissue, or in an aroma locket for this purpose. **Tip:** This blend is especially effective in helping individuals through the healing process from long-term stress and traumatic events.

Coping with Trauma- Blend #2:

1 drop rose absolute

1 drop geranium

1 drop benzoin

Inhale at 5-10 minute intervals throughout the day. Can be used in the palm of the hands, on a tissue, or in an aroma locket for this purpose. **Tip:** This blend is especially effective in helping women through the healing process

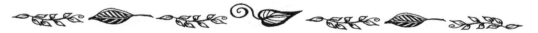

from past abuse, sexual assault, and uncomfortable feelings about self. Ideally used in conjunction with massage therapy.

Coping with Trauma- Blend #3:

2 drops pine needle

2 drops Atlas cedar

2 drops frankincense

1 drop spikenard

1 drop ylang ylang

Best inhaled and used in massage therapy with a focus of application on the adrenal area, the sacrum, solar plexus, and the heart center. **Tip:** This blend is especially effective in helping individuals through the healing process from traumatic events and accompanying anxiety.

Coping with Trauma- Blend #4:

2 drops pine needle

2 drops frankincense

2 drops sandalwood

1 drop juniper

Best used in massage therapy with a focus of application on the adrenal area, the sacrum, solar plexus, and the heart center. **Tip:** This blend is especially effective in helping individuals through the healing process from long-term stress and traumatic events.

Coping with Trauma- Blend #5:

2 drops frankincense

2 drops sandalwood

1 drop cypress

Best used in massage therapy with a focus of application on the adrenal area, the sacrum, solar plexus, and the heart center. **Tip:** This blend is especially effective in helping individuals through the healing process from traumatic loss/grief.

Coping with Trauma- Blend #6:

2 drops rose otto

2 drops benzoin

1 drop ylang ylang

1 drop tangerine

Best used in massage therapy with a focus of application on the adrenal area, the sacrum, solar plexus, and the heart center. **Tip:** This blend is especially effective in helping individuals through the healing process from childhood abuse or trauma.

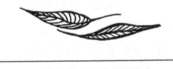

SELF-WORTH

Self-Worth/Confidence Blend #1:

1 drop allspice

1 drop sweet orange

1 drop vetiver

Inhale at 5-10 minute intervals throughout the day. Can be used in the palm of the hands, on a tissue, or in an aroma locket for this purpose.

Self-Worth/Confidence Blend #2:

1 drop juniper

1 drop lemon

1 drop cassia

Inhale at 5-10 minute intervals throughout the day. Can be on a tissue or in an aroma locket for this purpose.

Self-Worth/Confidence Blend #3:

1 drop ylang ylang

1 drop lemon

1 drop lemongrass

Inhale at 5-10 minute intervals throughout the day. Can be on a tissue or in an aroma locket for this purpose.

ANGER, RESENTMENT, FRUSTRATION

Anger Blend #1:

2 drops ylang ylang

1 drop neroli

1 drop lavender

Inhale at 5-10 minute intervals throughout the day. Can be used in the palm of the hands, on a tissue, or in an aroma locket for this purpose.

Anger Blend #2:

1 drop carrot seed

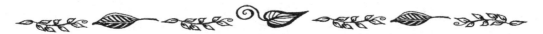

1 drop German chamomile

1 drop Roman chamomile

Inhale at 5-10 minute intervals throughout the day. Can be used in the palm of the hands, on a tissue, or in an aroma locket for this purpose. Can also be used in massage.

OBSESSIVE THOUGHTS OR PHOBIAS

Obsession Blend #1:

2 drops sweet orange

1 drop frankincense

Inhale at 5-10 minute intervals throughout the day. Can be used in the palm of the hands, on a tissue, or in an aroma locket for this purpose.

Obsession Blend #2:

2 drops pine needle

2 drops palo santo

Inhale at 5-10 minute intervals throughout the day. Can be used in the palm of the hands, on a tissue, or in an aroma locket for this purpose. **Tip:** This blend is especially effective for excessive worry.

Obsession Blend #3:

1 drop cinnamon leaf

1 drop basil

Inhale at 5-10 minute intervals throughout the day. Can be used on a tissue, or in an aroma locket for this purpose.

Obsession Blend #4:

2 drops neroli

1 drop sweet orange

Inhale at 5-10 minute intervals throughout the day. Can be used in the palm of the hands, on a tissue, or in an aroma locket for this purpose. **Tip:** This blend is especially effective for excessive worry.

NIGHTMARES

Nightmares Blend #1:

1 drop spikenard

1 drop Atlas cedar

1 drop lavender

Inhale at 5-10 minutes before bedtime and apply neat to the soles of the feet.

Nightmares Blend #2:

2 drops melissa

1 drop lavender

1 drop ylang ylang

Inhale at 5-10 minutes before bedtime and apply neat to the soles of the feet.

V

THERAPEUTIC STEAM INHALATION RECIPES

Colds/flu. Allergy symptoms. Sinus problems.

Respiratory congestion. Sore throat.

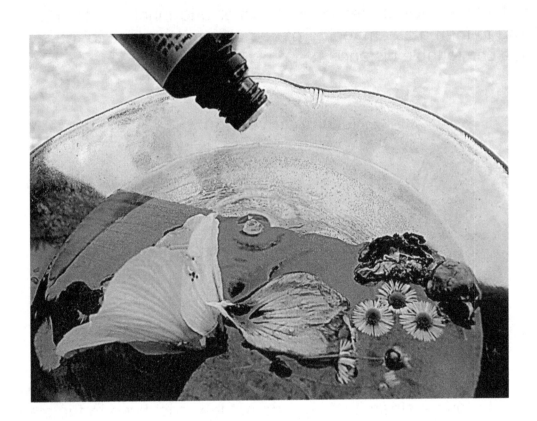

Cold/Flu Inhalation Blend #1:

2 drops peppermint

2 drops spearmint

2 drops juniper

2 drops pine needle

2 drops eucalyptus

dropped into a bowl of steaming-hot water and inhaled with a towel over the head to form a steam tent. <u>Tip</u>: do not lean too close to the steam and only at a comfortable distance.

Simpler version:

2 drops lemon eucalyptus

2 drops juniper

Cold/Flu Inhalation Blend #2:

2 drops juniper
2 drops spearmint
1 drop white thyme
1 drop wintergreen or sweet birch

dropped into a bowl of steaming-hot water and inhaled with a towel over the head to form a steam tent. <u>Tip</u>: do not lean too close to the steam and only at a comfortable distance.

Cold/Flu Inhalation Blend #3:

2 drops rosemary
2 drops balsam fir

dropped into a bowl of steaming-hot water and inhaled with a towel over the head to form a steam tent. <u>Tip</u>: do not lean too close to the steam and only at a comfortable distance.

Cold/Flu Inhalation Blend #4:

3 drops copaiba
3 drops frankincense
2 drops pine needle

dropped into a bowl of steaming-hot water and inhaled with a towel over the head to form a steam tent. <u>Tip</u>: do not lean too close to the steam and only at a comfortable distance.

This blend is especially useful for people who are asthmatic and/or cannot tolerate menthol.

Sore Throat Inhalation Blend #1

2 drops eucalyptus radiata
2 drops lime

dropped into a bowl of steaming-hot water and inhaled with a towel over the head to form a steam tent. <u>Tip</u>: do not lean too close to the steam and only at a comfortable distance.

Sore Throat Inhalation Blend #2

2 drops cajeput
1 drop tea tree
1 drop lemon

dropped into a bowl of steaming-hot water and inhaled with a towel over the head to form a steam tent. <u>Tip</u>: do not lean too close to the steam and only at a comfortable distance.

Sinus Support Inhalation Blend #1:

2 drops eucalyptus

3 drops pine needle

dropped into a bowl of steaming-hot water and inhaled with a towel over the head to form a steam tent. <u>Tip</u>: do not lean too close to the steam and only at a comfortable distance.

Sinus Support Inhalation Blend #2:

1 drop spearmint

1 drop lemon eucalyptus

3 drops juniper

dropped into a bowl of steaming-hot water and inhaled with a towel over the head to form a steam tent. <u>Tip</u>: do not lean too close to the steam and only at a comfortable distance.

Sinus Support Inhalation Blend #3:

4 drops pine needle

2 drops copaiba

dropped into a bowl of steaming-hot water and inhaled with a towel over the head to form a steam tent. <u>Tip</u>: do not lean too close to the steam and only at a comfortable distance.

This blend is especially useful for people who are asthmatic and/or cannot tolerate menthol.

Lung Congestion Inhalation Blend #1:

3 drops eucalyptus

3 drops balsam fir

dropped into a bowl of steaming-hot water and inhaled with a towel over the head to form a steam tent. <u>Tip</u>: do not lean too close to the steam and only at a comfortable distance.

Lung Congestion Inhalation Blend #2:

2 drops peppermint

1 drop lemon eucalyptus

1 drop lemongrass

dropped into a bowl of steaming-hot water and inhaled with a towel over the head to form a steam tent. <u>Tip</u>: do not lean too close to the steam and only at a comfortable distance.

Lung Congestion Inhalation Blend #3:

3 drops Peru balsam

2 drops frankincense

2 drops white fir, balsam fir, or pine needle

dropped into a bowl of steaming-hot water and inhaled with a towel over the head to form a steam tent. <u>Tip</u>: do not lean too close to the steam and only at a comfortable distance.

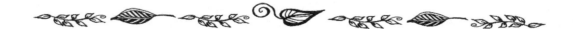

<u>VI</u>

THERAPEUTIC BATHS AND FOOTBATHS

Colds/flu. Stress reduction.

Pain management. Preparation for sleep

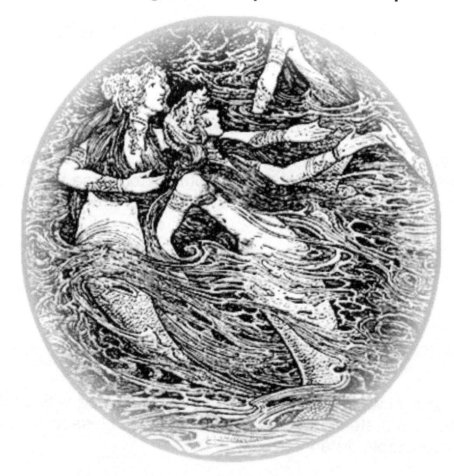

Basic Bath and Footbath Guidelines

One time use: Add essential oils to a base of ¼ cup Epsom salts and 1 tablespoon of evaporated sea salt or Himalayan pink salt and stir well. Fill tub or plastic basin/foot spa with warm-to-hot water according to tolerance level and add bath salts.

Larger batch: Add up to 50 drops essential oils to a base of 1 cup Epsom salts and 1/4 of evaporated sea salt or Himalayan pink salt and stir well. Store in an air-tight jelly or Mason jar. Use within 6 months for maximum potency.

THERAPEUTIC FOOTBATHS FOR WELLBEING

One-Time Use Footbath Blends

Stress Management Footbath #1:

4 drops balsam fir

2 drops juniper

2 drops basil

in ¼ cup Epsom salts with one tablespoon evaporated sea salt or Himalayan pink salt. Mix well and add to water. <u>Tip</u>: Especially effective in the morning or after a long day. Supports the adrenals and nervous system.

Stress Management Footbath #2:

5 drops lavender

2 drops geranium

in ¼ cup Epsom salts with one tablespoon evaporated sea salt or Himalayan pink salt. Mix well and add to water. <u>Tip</u>: Especially effective in after a long day. For overall wellbeing and balance.

Stress Management Footbath #3:

4 drops peppermint

3 drops pine needle

1 drop pine bark

in ¼ cup Epsom salts with one tablespoon evaporated sea salt or Himalayan pink salt. Mix well and add to water. <u>Tip</u>: *Especially effective in the morning or after a long day. Supports the adrenals.*

Stress Management Footbath #4:

4 drops ylang ylang

2 drops lavender

1 drop geranium

in ¼ cup Epsom salts with one tablespoon evaporated sea salt or Himalayan pink salt. Mix well and add to water. <u>Tip</u>: *Especially effective after a long day. Supports the nervous system.*

Stress Management Footbath #5:

4 drops balsam fir

2 drops frankincense

1 drop Atlas cedarwood

in ¼ cup Epsom salts with one tablespoon evaporated sea salt or Himalayan pink salt. Mix well and add to water. <u>Tip</u>: *Especially effective after a long day. Supports the nervous and endocrine systems.*

THERAPEUTIC BATHS

One-Time Use Bath Blends

Immune-Boosting Bath #1:

4 drops pine needle

2 drops lemon eucalyptus

3 drops juniper

in ¼ cup Epsom salts with one tablespoon evaporated sea salt or Himalayan pink salt. Mix well and add to water.

Immune-Boosting Bath #2:

4 drops pine needle

5 drops lemon eucalyptus

in ¼ cup Epsom salts with one tablespoon evaporated sea salt or Himalayan pink salt. Mix well and add to water.

Immune-Boosting Bath #3:

3 drops pine needle

3 drops balsam fir

3 drops juniper

in ¼ cup Epsom salts with one tablespoon evaporated sea salt or Himalayan pink salt. Mix well and add to water.

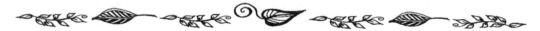

Immune-Boosting Bath #4:

4 drops juniper

1 drop ginger

in ¼ cup Epsom salts with one tablespoon evaporated sea salt or Himalayan pink salt. Mix well and add to water.

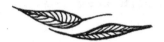

Relaxation Bath #1:

5 drops Roman chamomile
4 drops lavender
1 drop geranium or rose geranium
in ¼ cup Epsom salts with one tablespoon evaporated sea salt or Himalayan pink salt. Mix well and add to water.

Relaxation Bath #2:

4 drops ylang ylang

4 drops vetiver

in ¼ cup Epsom salts with one tablespoon evaporated sea salt or Himalayan pink salt. Mix well and add to water.

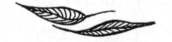

Restorative Bath #1:

4 drops balsam fir

3 drops black spruce

2 drops sweet marjoram

in ¼ cup Epsom salts with one tablespoon evaporated sea salt or Himalayan pink salt. Mix well and add to water. <u>Tip</u>: This is a wonderful bath for frayed nerves and low energy.

Restorative Bath #2:

5 drops pine needle

4 drops frankincense

1 drop cypress

in ¼ cup Epsom salts with one tablespoon evaporated sea salt or Himalayan pink salt. Mix well and add to water. <u>Tip</u>: This is a wonderful bath for frayed nerves and low energy.

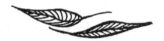

Women's Hormonal Support Bath #1:

4 drops clary sage

2 drops geranium

2 Roman chamomile

in ¼ cup Epsom salts with one tablespoon evaporated sea salt or Himalayan pink salt. Mix well and add to water.

Women's Hormonal Support Bath #2:

4 drops lavender

2 drops cypress

in ¼ cup Epsom salts with one tablespoon evaporated sea salt or Himalayan pink salt. Mix well and add to water.

Women's Hormonal Support Bath #3:

4 drops jasmine

2 drops Roman chamomile

1 drop ylang ylang

in ¼ cup Epsom salts with one tablespoon evaporated sea salt or Himalayan pink salt. Mix well and add to water.

Women's Hormonal Support Bath #4:

3 drops clary sage

2 drops spearmint

2 drops Roman chamomile

in ¼ cup Epsom salts with one tablespoon evaporated sea salt or Himalayan pink salt. Mix well and add to water.

Better Sleep Bath #1:

3 drops ylang ylang

3 drops rosewood

3 drops neroli

in ¼ cup Epsom salts with one tablespoon evaporated sea salt or Himalayan pink salt. Mix well and add to water. Tip: This is a wonderful bath before bed.

Better Sleep Bath #2:

3 drops balsam fir

3 drops rosewood

2 drops Atlas cedarwood

2 drops lavender

in ¼ cup Epsom salts with one tablespoon evaporated sea salt or Himalayan pink salt. Mix well and add to water. Tip: This is a wonderful bath before bed.

<u>VII</u>

RECIPES FOR THE HOUSEHOLD

All-purpose spray cleaners. Scrubbing powders. Room sprays.

Air fresheners. Potpourri. Mold eliminators. House plant health.

Pest repellant. Fragrant tips

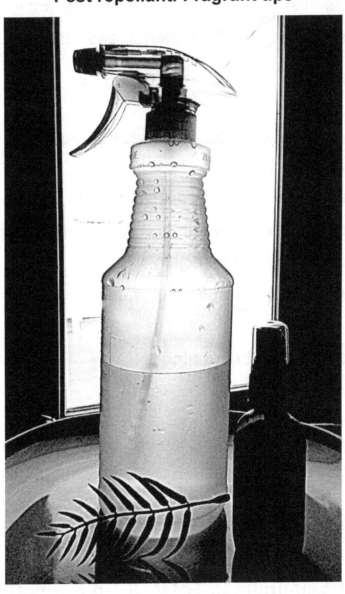

ALL-PURPOSE COUNTERTOP SPRAY CLEANERS

Cleaning with essential oils is delightful and healthier for us and the environment, and most of all, effective. The following spray cleaner recipes can be used in every room in the house and most surfaces except for fine wood. They are ideal for kitchen countertops, stoves, refrigerators, and tables and bathrooms. The following blends are antimicrobial, antiviral, antifungal, and antiseptic, smell wonderful, and offer all of their inhalation benefits.

Basic Guidelines for Spray Cleaners

Fill a large spray bottle ¾ full (available in dollar stores and retail stores in the cleaning or gardening department) with distilled water (found in any supermarket in the bottled water section)

Add approximately 50-60 drops of universal and other essential oils of choice

Add 2-3 tablespoons of rubbing alcohol

Shake well before use

Tip: Be sure to include a universal oil in heavy-duty spray cleaners to ensure a total cleaning effect **e.g.** lemon, clove, lavender, tea tree, white thyme, or lemon eucalyptus

RECIPES FOR ALL-PURPOSE SPRAY CLEANERS

Ginger-Lemongrass Total Clean Spray Cleaner:

30 drops lemongrass

30 drops lemon or organic lemon

10 drops ginger

2-3 tablespoons rubbing alcohol

added to spray bottle ¾ filled with distilled water. Shake well before use.

Basil-Peppermint-Eucalyptus Spray Cleaner:

30 drops peppermint

12 drops lemon eucalyptus

15 drops basil

2-3 tablespoons rubbing alcohol

added to spray bottle ¾ filled with distilled water. Shake well before use.

Lemon Forest Total Clean Spray Cleaner:

40 drops juniper

20 drops lemon or organic lemon

20 drops pine needle

2-3 tablespoons rubbing alcohol

added to spray bottle ¾ filled with distilled water. Shake well before use.

Lemon-Tea Tree Total Clean Spray Cleaner:

40 drops juniper

20 drops lemon or organic lemon

20 drops pine needle

2-3 tablespoons rubbing alcohol

added to spray bottle ¾ filled with distilled water. Shake well before use.

Sweet Lavender-Lemon Total Clean Spray Cleaner:

40 drops lavender

25 drops lemon or organic lemon

10 drops ylang ylang

2-3 tablespoons rubbing alcohol

added to spray bottle ¾ filled with distilled water. Shake well before use.

Spiced Coffee Total Clean Spray Cleaner:

25 drops clove

15 drops coffee bean

3 drops cardamom

2 drops nutmeg

2-3 tablespoons rubbing alcohol

added to spray bottle ¾ filled with distilled water. Shake well before use

Scented Geranium-Lavender Total Clean Spray Cleaner:

30 drops geranium or rose geranium

30 drops lavender

2-3 tablespoons rubbing alcohol

added to spray bottle ¾ filled with distilled water. Shake well before use.

Tangerine-Citrus Total Clean Spray Cleaner:

30 drops tangerine

25 drops grapefruit

20 drops lemon or organic lemon

2-3 tablespoons rubbing alcohol

added to spray bottle ¾ filled with distilled water. Shake well before use.

French Fields Total Clean Spray Cleaner:

20 drops lavender

15 drops white thyme

10 drops spearmint

3 drops rosemary

2-3 tablespoons rubbing alcohol

added to spray bottle ¾ filled with distilled water. Shake well before use.

Sweet Orange-Spice Total Clean Spray Cleaner:

35 drops sweet orange

20 drops clove

10 drops cassia

2-3 tablespoons rubbing alcohol

added to spray bottle ¾ filled with distilled water. Shake well before use.

Lavender-Lemongrass Total Clean Spray Cleaner:

30 drops lavender

20 drops lemongrass

2-3 tablespoons rubbing alcohol

added to spray bottle ¾ filled with distilled water. Shake well before use.

Forest Spice Total Clean Spray Cleaner:

30 drops balsam fir

20 drops clove

5 drops patchouli

2-3 tablespoons rubbing alcohol

added to spray bottle ¾ filled with distilled water. Shake well before use.

Rosemary-Lime Total Clean Spray Cleaner:

40 drops lime

20 drops lemon

5 drops rosemary

2-3 tablespoons rubbing alcohol

added to spray bottle ¾ filled with distilled water. Shake well before use.

Cinnamon Leaf-Lemon Total Clean Spray Cleaner:

30 drops cinnamon leaf

20 drops lemon

2-3 tablespoons rubbing alcohol

added to spray bottle ¾ filled with distilled water. Shake well before use.

Lemon-Anise Total Clean Spray Cleaner:

40 drops lemon

12 drops anise seed or star anise

2-3 tablespoons rubbing alcohol

added to spray bottle ¾ filled with distilled water. Shake well before use.

GLASS CLEANER

Lemon-Fresh Mirror and Glass Cleaner:

20 drops lemon

3-4 tablespoons rubbing alcohol

1 tablespoon white vinegar

added to spray bottle ¾ filled with distilled water. Shake well before use.

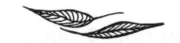

SCRUBBING POWDERS

Basic Guidelines for Scrubbing Powders

Add up to 50 drops of essential oil to 1 cup of baking soda, mix well and store in an air-tight Mason jar or other glass container. Use as you would any other scrubbing powder for tubs, counters, and sinks. Rinse well. <u>Tip</u>: Be cautious with certain sink and counter finishes; be sure baking soda is not too course.

Lemon-Tea Tree Total Clean Scrubbing Powder:

15 drops lemon or organic lemon

10 drops tea tree

1 drop spearmint

added to one cup baking soda

Lavender-Sweet Orange Total Clean Scrubbing Powder:

15 drops sweet orange

10 drops lavender

added to one cup baking soda

Spearmint-Lemon Eucalyptus Total Clean Scrubbing Powder:

8 drops spearmint

4 drops lemon eucalyptus

added to one cup baking soda

Grapefruit-Lemon Total Clean Scrubbing Powder:

10 drops lemon or organic lemon

10 drops grapefruit

added to one cup baking soda

Ginger-Lemongrass Total Clean Scrubbing Powder:

5 drops ginger

5 drops lemongrass

added to one cup baking soda

Balsam Fir-Clove Total Clean Scrubbing Powder:

10 drops balsam fir

6 drops clove

added to one cup baking soda

Spiced Coffee Total Clean Scrubbing Powder:

4 drops coffee bean

2 drops clove

1 drop nutmeg

1 drop cardamom

added to one cup baking soda

French Fields Total Clean Scrubbing Powder:

10 drops lavender

3 drops white thyme

2 drops rosemary

1 drop spearmint

added to one cup baking soda

Scented Geranium-Lavender Total Clean Scrubbing Powder:

10 drops lavender

5 drops geranium

added to one cup baking soda

COMBATING MOLD

Combine approximately 30 drops of essential oils per 1 cup of borax solution (borax and water) and wipe down area. This can also be made into a spray solution.

Mold-fighting essential oil combos:

tea tree / peppermint

tea tree / lavender

tea tree / eucalyptus

lemon eucalyptus / rosalina

tea tree / spike lavender / peppermint

tea tree / clove / eucalyptus

tea tree / rosemary

FRAGRANT ROOM SPRAYS TO SET THE MOOD

Basic Guidelines for Room Sprays

Fill a medium-large spritzer/spray bottle ¾ with distilled water and add approximately 60-70 drops of essential oils. Shake well.

Sweet Lavender Room Spray:

35 drops lavender

25 drops ylang ylang

added to distilled water in a spray bottle. Shake well.

Earl Grey-Citrus Room Spray:

30 drops bergamot

25 drops lemon

20 drops tangerine or sweet orange

added to distilled water in a spray bottle. Shake well.

Chocolate Lavender Room Spray:

30 drops cacao

15 drops lavender

12 drops ylang ylang

added to distilled water in a spray bottle. Shake well.

Lemongrass-Spearmint Room Spray:

30 drops lemongrass

25 drops spearmint

4 drops cinnamon leaf

added to distilled water in a spray bottle. Shake well.

Autumn Spice Room Spray:

20 drops clove

20 drops cassia

10 drops nutmeg

added to distilled water in a spray bottle. Shake well.

Pine-Patchouli Room Spray:

30 drops pine needle

20 drops balsam fir

15 drops patchouli

added to distilled water in a spray bottle. Shake well.

Sage-Cedar Room Spray:

50 drops Texas cedar

20 drops sage (Salvia officinalis)

added to distilled water in a spray bottle. Shake well.

Sweet Woods Room Spray:

40 drops palo santo

20 drops amrys

added to distilled water in a spray bottle. Shake well.

Sweet Floral Room Spray:

40 drops geranium

30 drops ylang ylang

added to distilled water in a spray bottle. Shake well.

EFFECTIVE AIR FRESHENERS

Basic Guidelines for Air Fresheners

Fill a medium-large spray bottle ¾ with distilled water and add approximately 40-60 drops of essential oils. Shake well. Can be used to clear the air in kitchens and bathrooms.

Forest Mint Air Freshener:

30 drops peppermint

15 drops balsam fir

10 drops pine needle

added to distilled water in a spray bottle. Shake well.

Lemon Anisette Air Freshener:

30 drops anise seed or star anise

25 drops lemon

added to distilled water in a spray bottle. Shake well.

Spicy Tangerine Air Freshener:

30 drops cassia

20 drops tangerine

10 drops cinnamon leaf

added to distilled water in a spray bottle. Shake well.

Ginger-Lemongrass Air Freshener:

30 drops lemongrass

8 drops ginger

added to distilled water in a spray bottle. Shake well.

Rosemary-Lavender Air Freshener:

30 drops lavender or spike lavender

20 drops rosemary

added to distilled water in a spray bottle. Shake well.

Key Lime Air Freshener:

30 drops lime

10 drops lemon

added to distilled water in a spray bottle. Shake well.

Sweet Mint-Cinnamon Leaf Air Freshener:

30 drops cinnamon leaf

8 drops spearmint

added to distilled water in a spray bottle. Shake well.

NATURAL POTPOURRIS

Creating custom-blended, natural potpourri is easy and enjoyable, and most of all, aromatherapeutic! Collect natural materials in the wild and/or from craft stores and choose some colorful additions such as mosses, lichen, dried red roses, and dried cedar berries. Choose your own essential oil combinations according to mood, season, and inspiration.

Basic Guidelines for Making Potpourri

Gather dried materials such as leaves, mosses, barks, flowers, rose petals, twigs, pine needles, rose hips, lichen, wild berries, etc. in a bowl, **add up to 25 drops or more of essential oil per cup of potpourri** and **stir gently** with a wooden spoon to distribute the oils. **Display** in a pretty

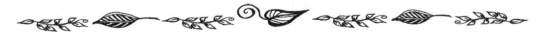

basket, cup, or bowl OR store in an air-tight decorative box. Refresh as desired.

ESSENTIAL OIL RECIPES FOR POTPOURRI

The following recipes are best as suggested but can certainly be adapted and simplified using only 2-3 essential oils on the list

> ### SUMMER INSPIRATIONS

<u>Sweet Summer Potpourri Blend</u>

8 drops ylang ylang

5 drops Roman chamomile

2 drops lavender

2 drops geranium

1 drop clary sage

added to dried natural materials and stirred gently to

distribute the essential oils

<u>Patio Herbs Potpourri Blend</u>

1 drop rosemary

2 drops Roman chamomile

1 drop basil

1 drop lavender

1 drop sweet marjoram

1 drop white thyme

1 drop spearmint

1 drop sage or clary sage

added to dried natural materials and stirred gently to

distribute the essential oils

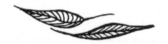

AUTUMN INSPIRATIONS

Autumn Garden Potpourri Blend

3 drops balsam fir

3 drops Peru balsam

3 drops amrys

2 drops clove

2 drops Texas cedar

1 drop nutmeg

1 drop tagetes

1 drop patchouli

added to dried natural materials and stirred gently to

distribute the essential oils

Turning Leaves Potpourri Blend

3 drops pine needle

2 drops sweet orange

2 drops benzoin

1 drop nutmeg

1 drop vetiver

added to dried natural materials and stirred gently to

distribute the essential oils

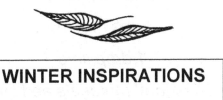

WINTER INSPIRATIONS

Morning Snow Potpourri Blend

20 drops pine needle

3 drops peppermint

added to dried natural materials and stirred gently to

distribute the essential oils

Winter Twilight Potpourri Blend

12 drops balsam fir

3 drops juniper

1 drop clove

added to dried natural materials and stirred gently to

distribute the essential oils

Spring Green Potpourri Blend

3 drops clary sage

3 drops bergamot

2 drops rosemary

1 drop lime

added to dried natural materials and stirred gently to

distribute the essential oils

April Breeze Potpourri Blend

4 drops ylang ylang

1 drop clary sage

1 drop peppermint

added to dried natural materials and stirred gently to

distribute the essential oils

DESERT INSPIRATIONS

Moroccan Moon Potpourri Blend

8 drops ylang ylang

5 drops frankincense

5 drops myrrh

5 drops amrys

5 drops benzoin

1 drop cardamom

1 drop coriander seed

added to dried natural materials and stirred gently to

distribute the essential oils

Sage Wind Potpourri Blend

15 dropsTexas cedar

5 drops juniper

4 drops sage (Salvia officinalis)

added to dried natural materials and stirred gently to

distribute the essential oils

DELICIOUS INSPIRATIONS

Mocha Bliss Potpourri Blend

15 drops cacao

5 drops coffee bean

4 drops Peru balsam

added to dried natural materials and stirred gently to

distribute the essential oils

Sweet Cinnamon Potpourri Blend

15 drops cassia

8 drops ylang ylang

1 drop clove

added to dried natural materials and stirred gently to

distribute the essential oils

Citrus Sorbet Potpourri Blend

15 drops tangerine

10 drops palmarosa

8 drops grapefruit

8 drops lemon

2 drops Peru balsam

added to dried natural materials and stirred gently to

distribute the essential oils

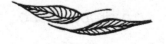

HOUSEHOLD PLANT HEALTH

To combat molds and fungus in the soil of house plants, add 2 drops rosewood and 2 drops tea tree essential oil to every cup of water used for watering and swirl to mix well. If the plant is already affected by harmful molds or fungus, use this water for a period of 4 weeks, even if there is evidence that the offender is under control. For healthy plants, use this water once a week or twice a month.

DETERRING SPIDERS
and OTHER PESTS

To deter spiders from entering through your doors and windows, fill a large spray bottle ¾ full with distilled water and add 60-80 drops of peppermint essential oil. Shake well before use and spray along doorframes (top, bottom, and sides) *outside and inside* and along window sills. Spray the floor *around all beds* including pet beds. Do this a couple times a week. Variation: To deter scorpions, add 60 drops lavender/10 drops peppermint.

FRAGRANT IDEAS

Rub your favorite essential oils on unscented candles (4-6 drops per candle) and allow to dry for about three hours before burning. Scented candles can be stored in an airtight box;
use within a week for freshness.

Use floating candles and scent the water (up to 10 drops of essential oils); sprinkle rose petals or other blooms in the water for a nice touch

Candle suggestions:

cacao (chocolate) / sweet orange

(use darker color candles- cacao will leave unsightly stains on lighter colors)

coffee bean / cacao (chocolate)
(use darker color candles for cacao will leave unsightly stains on lighter colors)

lavender / geranium

lemon / ylang ylang

lemongrass / ginger

balsam fir / clove /sweet orange

nutmeg / cassia / clove

FRAGRANT FIRES

Sprinkle 10-15 drops of essential oil onto logs and allow the oils to be absorbed into the wood for about an hour before you put them into the fireplace.

Suggested Combinations for Fragrant Fires:

balsam fir / juniper

cassia / clove

clove / pine needle

Texas cedar / sage

Texas cedar / juniper

nutmeg / cardamom

ginger / clove

palo santo / balsam fir

black spruce / pine bark

AIR CONDITIONING FILTERS

Sprinkle up to 8-10 drops of peppermint, lemongrass, spearmint, or lavender essential oil onto wall and window air conditioning units for a fresh scent and to combat mold and mildew in humid weather

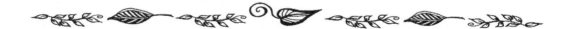

VIII

SYNERGISTIC BLENDS
FOR VIBRATIONAL AROMATIC THERAPY

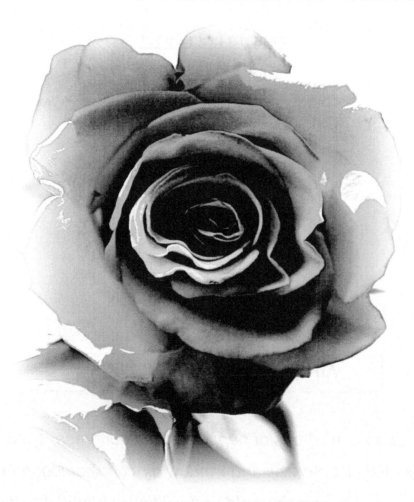

Energy medicine is no longer a "New Age" curiosity but a cutting-edge field led by scientists such as Jim Oschman and based upon the scientific basis of physics, biology, and chemistry.

Even *before* body chemistry exhibits imbalances that result in illness, *electromagnetic changes* alter cells and organs. Bringing these altered cells back into harmonic states leads to healing, and the use of essential oils can be a direct route. Oschman calls this work *energetic pharmacology* to differentiate it from chemical pharmacology. Since frequency changes with thought, emotion, mood, and atmospheric pressure, there is no certain constancy of reference for the vibratory rate of essential oils, but it can be said that each essential oil possesses frequency that ranges from 52-320 megahertz, and when applied to the body, will raise the vibratory rate of the individual. In essence, this process is *harmonic resonance at the subatomic level*. Chemical pharmaceutical medications possess zero frequency which means no life force.

Using essential oils to raise the body's frequency may have a profound effect on molecular integrity and contribute to a healthier life. The physical body vibrates between 62 and 68 MHz. Cell mutations begin when the frequency drops below 62 MHZ. Colds and influenza thrive when the body drops to 58 MHz, cancer around 42 MHz. The human energy or auric field is an electromagnetic mote of sorts, emitting light and color (energy). When our energy field is weak, our immune systems are usually compromised and vice versa. Pathogens both physical and energetic can easily invade the body and spirit, weakening our reserves and life force. Essential oils help keep our physical bodies and auric shields more vital even when we are exposed to microbes, negative work or home environments, and insidious parasitic energies. One does not need to be 'spiritual' or religious in order to use or receive the benefits of vibrational aromatherapy, but positive thoughts, prayer, and Reiki have been shown to raise the frequency of essential oils by as much as 15 MHz while negative or agitated thoughts can lower their frequency by 12 MHz.

It is recommended that you approach essential oil applications with a

serene and untroubled state of mind as much as possible in order to reap the maximum benefits. Vibrational aromatherapy also can be used to raise the energy level of living spaces and to clear areas of accumulated emotional imprints.

The following recipes suggest essential oils of higher frequency and those that have a specific effect when combined with each other. They can be used to reestablish harmony in the energy field after spending long hours on the job, in a large group of people, or draining atmospheres such as work environments that involve high-stress levels, illness (hospitals) or anywhere our energies are compromised and sapped. Using vibrational applications during stressful and difficult times helps us weather the storm better on the cellular level. Situations that involve caregiving, someone struggling with addiction, working with negative people, losing someone through separation or death, or recovering from illness are all appropriate times to use essential oils for building up energetic reserves. Making it a daily habit also is a wonderful way to build and maintain these precious reserves.

The Energy or Auric Field – a Brief Overview

The Etheric Field=closest to the physical body extending 2-4 inches outward. It is seen as an energetic double of the physical person.

The Emotional Field=where our emotions are stored and extends 8-20 inches outward from the physical body. Anger and grief are prominent emotions within this energy layer.

The Mental Field=the energy layer that vibrates quicker than the etheric and emotional and houses higher thought and creativity, extending 12-24 inches from the body, especially around the head.

The Spiritual Field or Spiritual Body=thought to be the layer that holds higher or essential consciousness, what is termed as the 'soul.' It can also be described as the source of inner knowing, inner truth, or the 'higher self.'

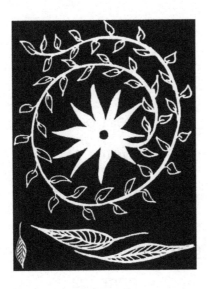

Recommended Essential Oils for:

<u>Strengthening the Energy Field</u>

Atlas cedarwood

black spruce

cypress

frankincense

galbanum

geranium

juniper

lavender

myrrh

nutmeg

palo santo

patchouli

pine bark

pine needle

rose

rosewood

sandalwood

sweet birch

vetiver

yarrow, blue

Cleansing the Energy Field

angelica

balsam fir

basil

cedar, Texas

chamomile, Roman

cinnamon leaf

eucalyptus

grapefruit

hyssop

jasmine

juniper

lavender

lavender, spike

lemon

niaouli

neroli

palmarosa

palo santo

peppermint

rose

spearmint

sweet birch

white fir

yarrow, blue

ylang ylang

COMBINATIONS FOR STRENGTHENING THE ENERGY FIELD

Strong Energy Field Blend #1:

3 drops frankincense

3 drops pine needle

apply neat to the soles of the feet or 1 drop of each essential oil to the

palms of the hands and comb the air around the body,

brushing limbs with gentle, sweeping motions

Strong Energy Field Blend #2:

2 drops basil

2 drops lavender

apply neat to the soles of the feet or 1 drop of each essential oil to the

palms of the hands and comb the air around the body,

brushing limbs with gentle, sweeping motions

Strong Energy Field Blend #3:

2 drops geranium

2 drops rose absolute

1 drop frankincense

apply neat to the soles of the feet or 1 drop of each essential oil to the

palms of the hands and comb the air around the body,

brushing limbs with gentle, sweeping motions

Strong Energy Field Blend #4:

2 drops palo santo

1 drop cypress

1 drop vetiver

apply neat to the soles of the feet or 1 drop of each essential oil to the

palms of the hands and comb the air around the body,

brushing limbs with gentle, sweeping motions

Strong Energy Field Blend #5:

2 drops myrrh

2 drops pine bark

1 drop Atlas cedarwood

apply neat to the soles of the feet or 1 drop of each essential oil to the

palms of the hands and comb the air around the body,

brushing limbs with gentle, sweeping motions

Strong Energy Field Blend #6:

2 drops black spruce

2 drops frankincense

apply neat to the soles of the feet or 1 drop of each essential oil to the

palms of the hands and comb the air around the body,

brushing limbs with gentle, sweeping motions

Strong Energy Field Blend #7:

2 drops rosewood

1 drop angelica root

apply neat to the soles of the feet or 1 drop of each essential oil to the

palms of the hands and comb the air around the body,

brushing limbs with gentle, sweeping motions

COMBINATIONS FOR CLEANSING THE ENERGY FIELD

Clean Energy Field Blend #1:

2 drops juniper

1 drop peppermint

apply neat to the soles of the feet or 1 drop of each essential oil to the

palms of the hands and comb the air around the body,

brushing limbs with gentle, sweeping motions

Clean Energy Field Blend #2:

2 drops Texas cedar

1 drop clary sage

apply neat to the soles of the feet or 1 drop of each essential oil to the

palms of the hands and comb the air around the body,

brushing limbs with gentle, sweeping motions

Clean Energy Field Blend #3:

2 drops lemon

1 drop basil

apply neat to the soles of the feet or 1 drop of each essential oil to the

palms of the hands and comb the air around the body,

brushing limbs with gentle, sweeping motions

Clean Energy Field Blend #4:

2 drops spearmint

1 drop cinnamon leaf

apply neat to the soles of the feet or 1 drop of each essential oil to the

palms of the hands and comb the air around the body,

brushing limbs with gentle, sweeping motions

Clean Energy Field Blend #5:

2 drops lemongrass

1 drop peppermint

apply neat to the soles of the feet or 1 drop of each essential oil to the

palms of the hands and comb the air around the body,

brushing limbs with gentle, sweeping motions

Clean Energy Field Blend #6:

2 drops Roman chamomile

1 drop lavender

apply neat to the soles of the feet or 1 drop of each essential oil to the

palms of the hands and comb the air around the body,

brushing limbs with gentle, sweeping motions

Clean Energy Field Blend #7:

2 drops angelica

1 drop ylang ylang

1 drop clove

apply neat to the soles of the feet or 1 drop of each essential oil to the

palms of the hands and comb the air around the body,

brushing limbs with gentle, sweeping motions

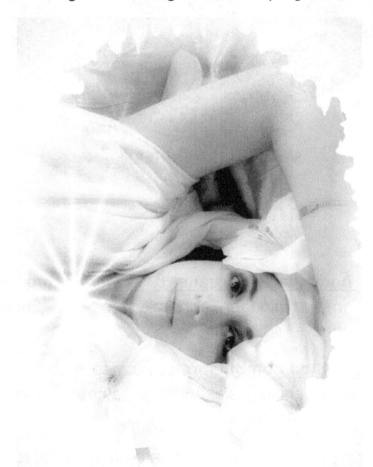

Chakras within the Energetic Network

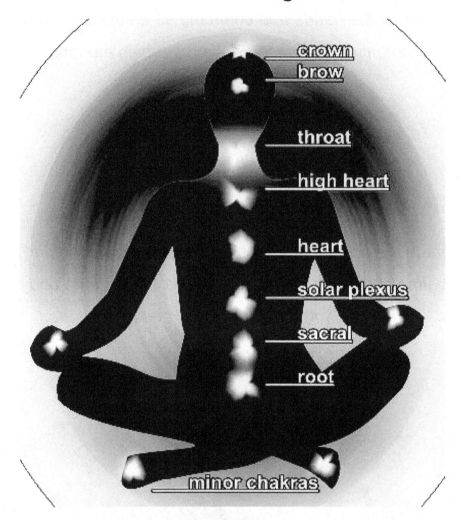

ROOT

location: coccyx

corresponding body parts, organs & systems: organs of excretion including the colon and bladder, adrenals, legs, hips, and lower back / excretory and immune

suggested essential oil combinations: nutmeg & vetiver / ginger & pine bark / patchouli & balsam fir / spikenard & patchouli / clove & patchouli / juniper berry & cypress / tsuga-vetiver

applications: apply diluted to the lower sacrum and neat to the soles of the feet

SACRAL a.k.a. the navel chakra

location: sacrum & first lumbar

corresponding body parts, organs & systems: organs of reproduction, large intestine / reproductive and excretory

suggested essential oil combinations: angelica & ylang ylang / geranium & vitex / jasmine & sweet orange / German chamomile & geranium / clove & ginger / angelica & vetiver

applications: apply diluted to the sacrum, lower back, and lower abdomen (1-2 inches below the belly button) and neat to the soles of the feet

SOLAR PLEXUS

location: solar plexus-upper abdomen

corresponding body parts, organs, & systems: pancreas, stomach, liver, gallbladder, adrenals, spleen, small intestine-transverse colon / gastrointestinal and endocrine systems

suggested essential oil combinations: Roman chamomile & neroli / peppermint & juniper berry / davana & lemon / sweet fennel & coriander / goldenrod & carrot seed / myrrh & balsam fir / frankincense & lemon / frankincense & Atlas cedarwood

applications: apply diluted to the abdomen and middle back

HEART

location: sternum- between the breasts

corresponding body parts, organs & systems: heart, lungs, shoulders, upper back / cardiovascular-circulatory and respiratory systems

suggested essential oil combinations: cardamom & cacao / rose & vanilla absolutes / geranium & rose absolute / benzoin & ylang ylang /

sweet marjoram & lavender / lavender & rose absolute / melissa & rose geranium

applications: apply diluted to the sternum and middle-upper back and neat to the soles of the feet

HIGH HEART a.k.a. the thymic chakra

location: between the sternum and throat

corresponding body parts, organs & systems: thymus / immune system

suggested essential oil combinations: lemon eucalyptus & geranium / clary sage & spearmint / hyssop & anise seed / benzoin & rose absolute / myrrh & benzoin

applications: upper chest

THROAT

location: throat-back of neck

corresponding organs & systems: thyroid, teeth, and neck

suggested essential oil combinations: clary sage & anise seed / eucalyptus & peppermint / blue yarrow & lavender / goldenrod & German chamomile / Peru balsam & pine needle

applications: apply diluted to the throat area and the back of the neck

BROW

location: between the eyebrows, middle of forehead

corresponding organs & systems: brain, especially the pineal and pituitary glands; eyes, nose, ears, sinuses / endocrine, lymphatic, and nervous systems

suggested essential oil combinations: Australian blue cypress & blue yarrow / Atlas cedar & spikenard / sandalwood & rose / myrrh & amrys / lavender & German chamomile / clary sage & lemongrass

applications: apply diluted in small amounts to middle of forehead

CROWN

location: top of the head with connection along the spinal cord

corresponding organs & systems: all

suggested essential oil combinations: sandalwood & jasmine / sandalwood & rose / frankincense & myrrh / rose & jasmine absolutes / white lotus & sandalwood / ylang ylang & sandalwood

applications: from the base of the skull to the coccyx all along the spine

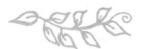

THE ENERGY OF PHYSICAL SPACES

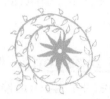

SPACE-CLEARING ROOM SPRAYS

Vibrational room sprays are an excellent way to disperse dense energies, consecrate new living spaces, and clear the air to restore harmony.

Recommended Essential Oils for Space Clearing

anise seed or star anise

balsam fir

basil

cinnamon leaf

clary sage

clove

cypress

cypress, blue

frankincense

jasmine

juniper berry

lavender

lemon

lemongrass

myrrh

palo santo

peppermint

pine needle

rose

rosemary

sage

spearmint

sweet birch

sweet marjoram

white fir

yarrow, blue

ylang ylang

Basic Guidelines for Space-Clearing Room Sprays

Fill a medium-large spritzer/spray bottle ¾ with distilled water and add approximately 60-70 drops of essential oils. Shake well.

Space-Clearing Room Spray #1:

35 drops palo santo

25 drops balsam fir

added to distilled water in a spray bottle. Shake well.

Space-Clearing Room Spray #2:

35 drops peppermint

25 drops juniper berry

added to distilled water in a spray bottle. Shake well.

Space-Clearing Room Spray #3:

20 drops blue yarrow

20 drops clary sage

added to distilled water in a spray bottle. Shake well.

Space-Clearing Room Spray #4:

30 drops Texas cedar

20 drops sage (Salvia officinalis)

10 drops juniper berry

added to distilled water in a spray bottle. Shake well.

Space-Clearing Room Spray #5:

30 drops lavender or spike lavender

20 drops ylang ylang

15 drops lemon

added to distilled water in a spray bottle. Shake well.

Space-Clearing Room Spray #6:

30 drops pine needle

15 drops rosemary

added to distilled water in a spray bottle. Shake well.

Space-Clearing Room Spray #7:

30 drops pre-diluted Roman chamomile

6 drops lemongrass

added to distilled water in a spray bottle. Shake well.

Space-Clearing Room Spray #8:

30 drops pine needle

10 drops sweet birch

added to distilled water in a spray bottle. Shake well.

Space-Clearing Room Spray #9:

30 drops pre-diluted rose

10 drops myrrh

10 drops frankincense

added to distilled water in a spray bottle. Shake well.

Space-Clearing Room Spray #10:

25 drops anise or star anise

20 drops lemon

added to distilled water in a spray bottle. Shake well.

Space-Clearing Room Spray #11:

25 drops sweet marjoram

20 drops spearmint

added to distilled water in a spray bottle. Shake well.

<u>IX</u>

ESSENTIAL BODY CARE

Luxurious Baths. Body spritzers. Dusting powders.

Body scrubs. Facial masks. Lip treatments. Mouthwash

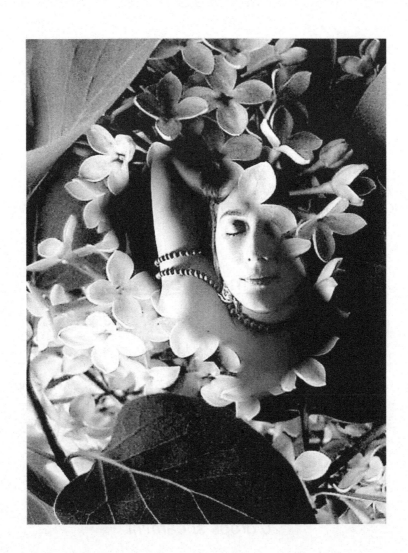

LUXURIOUS BATHS

Basic Bath and Footbath Guidelines

One time use: Add 4-12 drops of essential oils to a base of ¼ cup Epsom salts and 1 tablespoon of evaporated sea salt or Himalayan pink salt and stir well. Fill tub or plastic basin/foot spa with warm-to-hot water according to tolerance level and add bath salts.

Larger batch: Add up to 50 drops essential oils to a base of 1 cup Epsom salts and 1/4 of evaporated sea salt or Himalayan pink salt and stir well. Store in an air-tight jelly or Mason jar. Use within 6 months for potency.

One-Time Use Luxurious Bath Blends

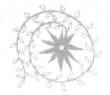

Chocolate and Flowers Bath Crystals:

8 drops cacao

3 drops ylang ylang

3 drops lavender

¼ cup dried rose petals (optional)

in ¼ cup Epsom salts with one tablespoon evaporated sea salt or Himalayan pink salt. Mix well and add to water.

In the Garden of Aphrodite Bath Crystals

7 drops ylang ylang

4 drops jasmine absolute or pre-diluted jasmine

4 drops rose absolute or pre-diluted rose

¼ cup dried rose petals or dried jasmine blooms (optional)

in ¼ cup Epsom salts with one tablespoon evaporated sea salt or Himalayan pink salt. Mix well and add to water.

Wood Nymph Bath Crystals

6 drops pine needle

4 drops vetiver

4 drops black spruce or white fir

in ¼ cup Epsom salts with one tablespoon evaporated sea salt or Himalayan pink salt. Mix well and add to water.

Temple Incense Bath Crystals

8 drops amrys

2 drops cardamom

3 drops ylang ylang

in ¼ cup Epsom salts with one tablespoon evaporated sea salt or Himalayan pink salt. Mix well and add to water.

Basic Face and Body Scrub Guidelines

Add 3-5 drops essential oils and ½ tablespoon extra virgin olive oil to 1 cup white or brown sugar. Mix well and store in an air-tight Mason jar. Use within 3 months for potency. **Variation:** Add ½ tablespoon of fine-textured evaporated sea salt or Himalayan pink salt to the mixture and blend well.

Tip: Turbinado sugar is not recommended, for it is a courser texture that could irritate the skin when used as a scrub.

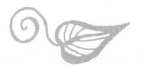

Cocoa Brown Sugar Scrub

3 drops cacao essential oil

½ tablespoon extra virgin olive oil

added to ¾ cup brown sugar and 2 tablespoons of cocoa powder. Mix well and store in a glass Mason jar. **To use:** Scoop desired amount into hand and scrub face and body in circular motions. Rinse with warm-hot water.

Lavender Sugar Scrub

3 drops lavender essential oil

½ tablespoon extra virgin olive oil

added to ¾ cup sugar. Mix well and store in a glass Mason jar. **To use:** Scoop desired amount into hand and scrub face and body in circular motions. Rinse with warm-hot water. **Variation:** Add a tablespoon of dried

lavender flowers to the mixture for pretty color and added exfoliating texture.

Geranium-Rose Brown Sugar Scrub

3 drops rose absolute or pre-diluted rose

1 drop geranium or rose geranium essential oil

½ tablespoon extra virgin olive oil

added to ¾ cup brown sugar. Mix well and store in a glass Mason jar. **To use:** Scoop desired amount into hand and scrub face and body in circular motions. Rinse with warm-hot water.

Herbal Sugar Scrub

4 drops Roman chamomile essential oil

1 drop lavender essential oil

½ tablespoon extra virgin olive oil

added to ¾ cup brown sugar. Mix well and store in a glass Mason jar. **To use:** Scoop desired amount into hand and scrub face and body in circular motions. Rinse with warm-hot water.

Vanilla-Mocha Brown Sugar Scrub

3 drops cacao essential oil

1 drop coffee bean essential oil

2 drops vanilla absolute or culinary vanilla extract

½ tablespoon extra virgin olive oil

added to ¾ cup brown sugar. Mix well and store in a glass Mason jar. **To use:** Scoop desired amount into hand and scrub face and body in circular motions. Rinse with warm-hot water.

PAMPERING FACIAL MASKS

These facial recipes use French green clay, but this can easily be substituted with food-grade bentonite clay (recommended for most skin types) or red Moroccan clay (a.k.a. Rhassoul clay & recommended for oily skin)

Chamomile-Orange Blossom Green Clay Mask

1 drop Roman chamomile essential oil

1 drop neroli essential oil

approx.1 teaspoon culinary orange blossom or rose water

added 1 tablespoon French green clay powder. Mix well into a paste and use immediately. If you'd like a thicker or thinner mask, add more clay or flower water for the desired consistency. **To use:** Apply to face and leave on for 15-20 minutes. Rinse gently with warm water or remove with a soft wash cloth and warm water. Finish with a splash of cool water. **Tip:** For dry or mature skin, add ¼ teaspoon of extra virgin olive oil to the mixture and blend well.

Chocolate and Roses Green Clay Mask

1 drop rose absolute or pre-diluted

approx.1 teaspoon culinary rose water

added to 1 teaspoon of pure cocoa powder and ¾ tablespoon of French green clay powder. Mix well into a paste and use immediately. If you'd like a thicker or thinner mask, add more clay or flower water for the desired consistency. **To use:** Apply to face and leave on for 15-20 minutes. Rinse gently with warm water or remove with a soft wash cloth and warm water. Finish with a splash of cool water. **Tip:** For dry or mature skin, add ¼ teaspoon of extra virgin olive oil to the mixture and blend well.

<u>Frankincense and Rose Green Clay Mask</u>

1 drop rose absolute or pre-diluted rose

1 drop frankincense essential oil

approx.1 teaspoon culinary rose water

added 1 tablespoon French green clay powder. Mix well into a paste and use immediately. If you'd like a thicker or thinner mask, add more clay or flower water for the desired consistency. **To use:** Apply to face and leave on for 15-20 minutes. Rinse gently with warm water or remove with a soft wash cloth and warm water. Finish with a splash of cool water. **Tip:** For dry or mature skin, add ¼ teaspoon of extra virgin olive oil to the mixture and blend well.

<u>Mermaid's Deep Clean Sea Kelp and Green Clay Mask</u>

1 drop clary sage essential oil

approx.1 teaspoon spring or tap water

added ½ tablespoon French green clay powder. and ½ tablespoon kelp granules or kelp powder. Mix well into a paste and use immediately. If you'd like a thicker or thinner mask, add more clay or water for the desired consistency. **To use:** Apply to face and leave on for 15-20 minutes. Rinse gently with warm water or remove with a soft wash cloth and warm water. Finish with a splash of cool water.

FRAGRANT BODY SPRITZERS

Basic Body Spritzer Guidelines

Fill a medium-sized spray/spritzer bottle (available in drug stores and

beauty supply outlets) **¾ full with distilled water** or culinary **rosewater** and **add approx. 30-50 drops of essential oils**. Shake well and spray all over body and hair, avoiding the eyes and face. **Tip:** Store body spritzers in the fridge during summer months for a refreshing skin treat.

Spicy Patchouli Body Spritzer

40 drops patchouli

2 drops clove

added to distilled water in a spritzer bottle. Shake well before use.

Tip: Makes a nice unisex body spray.

Sweet Lavender-Geranium Body Spritzer

15 drops lavender

10 drops ylang ylang

5 drops geranium

added to distilled water in a spritzer bottle. Shake well before use.

Orange Blossom-Bergamot Body Spritzer

25 drops neroli

10 drops bergamot

5 drops ylang ylang

added to distilled water or culinary orange blossom water in a spritzer bottle. Shake well before use.

Sweet Mocha Body Spritzer

20 drops cacao

6 drops coffee bean

5 drops ylang ylang

added to distilled water in a spritzer bottle. Shake well before use.

Tip: Makes a nice unisex body spray.

Earth and Forest Body Spritzer

20 drops pine needle

6 drops vetiver

added to distilled water in a spritzer bottle. Shake well before use.

Tip: Makes a nice unisex body spray.

Jasmine-Chamomile Body Spritzer

20 drops Roman chamomile

10 drops jasmine absolute or diluted jasmine

added to distilled water in a spritzer bottle. Shake well before use.

Winter Solstice Body Spritzer

15 drops balsam fir

5 drops frankincense

5 drops sweet orange

1 drop clove

added to distilled water in a spritzer bottle. Shake well before use.

Tip: Makes a nice unisex body spray.

Bay Rum Body Spritzer

10 drops bay (Pimenta racemosa)

1 drop clove

added to distilled water in a spritzer bottle. Shake well before use.

Tip: Makes a nice unisex body spray.

Ginger Flower Body Spritzer

20 drops ylang ylang

8 drops angelica root

2 drops ginger

added to distilled water in a spritzer bottle. Shake well before use.

Happiness Body Spritzer

10 drops bergamot

8 drops lavender

added to culinary rose water in a spritzer bottle. Shake well before use.

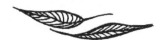

Basic Guidelines for Dusting Powders

Add up to 15 drops of essential oil to 1 cup of pure corn starch in a bowl. **Stir very well with a fork**, flattening each bead of essential oil until it dissolves into the corn starch.

Funnel into a grated cheese shaker and cover tightly. Cheese shakers can be found in any kitchen section of department stores or craft stores. Tip: The easiest and most convenient funnel to use is one

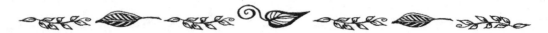

made of paper, curled around and adjusted to the opening of the jar/shaker.

Place a small strip of clear packaging tape over the holes and seal after each use. Powder can be used on the body and sprinkled in shoes for freshness. <u>Note:</u> Body powders with essential oils are not recommended for use on the face.

Morning Snow Dusting Powder

5 drops peppermint

4 drops pine needle

mixed well with 1 cup pure corn starch

Tip: Makes a nice unisex body powder.

Chocolate-Lavender Dusting Powder

10 drops cacao

4 drops lavender

mixed well with 1 cup pure corn starch

Chocolate and Roses Dusting Powder

10 drops cacao

6 drops rose absolute or pre-diluted rose

mixed well with 1 cup pure corn starch

Sahara Deodorizing Dusting Powder

10 drops myrrh

4 drops frankincense

3 drops ylang ylang

mixed well with 1 cup pure corn starch

Tip: Makes a nice unisex body powder.

Lavender Dusting Powder

10 drops lavender

mixed well with 1 cup pure corn starch

Tip: Makes a nice unisex body powder.

Jasmine-Orange Blossom Dusting Powder

10 drops neroli

8 drops jasmine absolute or pre-diluted jasmine

mixed well with 1 cup pure corn starch

Patchouli Deodorizing Dusting Powder

10 drops patchouli

mixed well with 1 cup pure corn starch

Tip: Makes a nice unisex body powder.

Scented Geranium Deodorizing Dusting Powder

6 drops geranium

2 drops ylang ylang

mixed well with 1 cup pure corn starch

Bay Rum-Spice Dusting Powder

7 drops bay (Pimenta racemosa)

1 drop clove mixed well with 1 cup pure corn starch

Tip: Makes a nice body powder for men.

Bay Rum-Patchouli Dusting Powder

7 drops bay (Pimenta racemosa)

5 drops patchouli

mixed well with 1 cup pure corn starch

Tip: Makes a nice body powder for men.

Angelica-Musk Dusting Powder

8 drops angelica root or pre-diluted angelica

7 drops amrys

mixed well with 1 cup pure corn starch

Tip: Makes a nice unisex body powder.

AROMATHERAPEUTIC

HONEY LIP TREATMENTS

This treatment can be used once a week to revive and plump the lips. It can be stored in an airtight glass container or wide-neck jar. Regular honey can be substituted for raw honey.

Grapefruit and Honey Lip Quencher

1 drop grapefruit essential oil

308

mixed well into 2 tablespoons raw honey. Store in a small glass container/jar. **Directions:** Apply a small amount to lips and leave on for 10 minutes. Rinse with warm water.

Chocolate and Honey Lip Quencher

1 drop cacao essential oil
mixed well into 2 tablespoons raw honey. Store in a small glass container/jar. **Directions:** Apply a small amount to lips and leave on for 10 minutes. Rinse with warm water.

Chamomile and Honey Lip Quencher

1 drop Roman chamomile essential oil
mixed well into 2 tablespoons raw honey. Store in a small glass container/jar. **Directions:** Apply a small amount to lips and leave on for 10 minutes. Rinse with warm water.

Lavender and Honey Lip Quencher

1 drop lavender essential oil
mixed well into 2 tablespoons raw honey. Store in a small glass container/jar. **Directions:** Apply a small amount to lips and leave on for 10 minutes. Rinse with warm water.

Rose and Honey Lip Quencher

1 drop rose absolute or pre-diluted rose
mixed well into 2 tablespoons raw honey. Store in a small glass container/jar. **Directions:** Apply a small amount to lips and leave on for 10 minutes. Rinse with warm water.

Daily Mouthwash #1

1 drop eucalyptus globulus

1 drop clove

1 drop peppermint

added to a 4 ounce cup then fill halfway with *warm* tap water and quickly swirl water in circular motions to mix the oils. Use as any other mouthwash, rinsing for 30-60 seconds before spitting out. Best used after brushing.
Tip: This is an excellent and refreshing mouthwash to combat mouth germs, plaque, gingivitis, and food odors. Use up to 3x a day.

Daily Mouthwash #2

1 drop lemongrass

1 drop spearmint

add to a 4 ounce cup then fill halfway with *warm* tap water and quickly swirl water in circular motions to mix the oils. Use as any other mouthwash, rinsing for 30-60 seconds before spitting out. Best used after brushing.
Tip: This is an excellent mouthwash to combat mouth germs, plaque, and gingivitis. Use up to 3x a day. This makes a very pleasant and effective mouthwash to combat mouth germs and bad breath.
Use up to 3x a day.

Healing Mouth Rinse

2 drops myrrh

¼ teaspoon of evaporated sea salt or Himalayan pink salt
add to a 4 ounce cup then fill halfway with *warm* tap water and quickly swirl water in circular motions to mix the oils. Use as any other mouthwash, rinsing for 60 seconds before spitting out.

Tip: This is a highly effective mouthwash to help heal mouth sores, inflamed gums or tissue, or after dental work.
Use up to 3x a day or as needed.

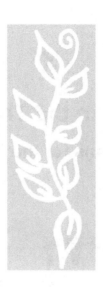

X

Essential Oils in the Treatment Room

Session Recommendations for the Professional Bodyworker

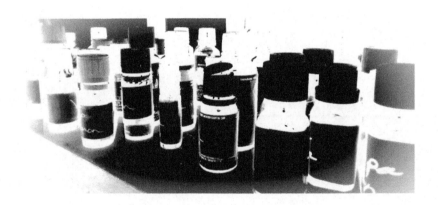

Using essential oils in bodywork can simply enhance any massage modality or be a strong component in the work. Having a good aromatherapy background can help you offer your clients many benefits of essential oils including:

lessen a client's soreness from post-deep tissue work by using essential oils during the massage session

encourage the client's sympathetic nervous system to yield to parasympathetic dominance and nurture stillpoint

enhance the benefits of massage and other modalities in cases of chronic pain syndromes

help athletes to experience quicker recovery after injury or strain

help ease a client through emotional sessions on the table

bring more oxygen to the tissues

introduce clients to the world of essential oil therapy who may have preconceived ideas about the practice

tailor sessions for multidimensional effects (body, mind, spirit)

experience more stamina, deeper concentration, and a stronger energy field as a bodyworker; excellent for long work days and many clients

Template for Aromatherapy Massage Sessions

1. **Determine which oils to use.** After accessing the client's intake form, discuss which oils might be of use during the session, keeping in mind contraindications, medications, and allergies/sensitivities.

2. **Breathe deeply.** Open the session by putting a drop or two in the palms of your hands; if the client is supine, cup your hands approximately six inches from the face while the client breathes in deeply for a minute or two; if the client is prone, cup your hands beneath the face cradle.

3. **Clear the energy field.** Put another drop or two of desired essential oil on the palms of your hands and make gentle, sweeping motions over the client's entire body as if combing the air. Clearing the client's energy field opens the door to receiving the maximum benefits of both massage and essential oils.

4. **Apply essential oils to the soles of the feet.** Apply a few drops of desired essential oil neat to the soles of the client's feet and gently cover them with the sheet or a towel beneath the sheet for extra warmth and easy absorption.

5. **Nourish the spine and sacrum.** When the client is prone, apply desired essential oils along the spine, beginning at the sacrum and working gently into the lamina grooves as you move upward to the neck; this is especially nourishing to the nervous system. **Recommended essential oils:** *rosewood, frankincense, ylang ylang, lavender, Roman chamomile*

6. **Use essential oils for specific work.** When doing deep or specific work, use a drop of spearmint, pine needle, lavender, or peppermint as you work the tissue to prevent client's post-massage soreness and to minimize your own

7. **Close with an auric cleanse.** At the conclusion of the session, gently cleanse the client's energy field once again, using gentle

sweeps over the body; this establishes equilibrium if any intense emotions (obvious or not) surfaced during the session.

8. **Clear your own energy field.** After the client leaves, you might consider putting a drop of peppermint or lavender in the palms of your hands to clear your own energy field by combing the air around your head, arms, torso, legs, and feet

9. **Clear the space.** At the end of the work day, you might consider misting the air with a space-clearing spray.

Essential Oil Combination Templates

Deep tissue aromatherapy massage template #1

Opening inhalation: 1 drop spearmint

Clearing the field: 1 drop lemongrass

Soles of the feet: 2 drops pine needle per foot

Along the spine/sacrum: 2 drops peppermint

Specific work: 1 drop spearmint

Closing oil: 1 drop lemongrass

......

Deep tissue aromatherapy massage template #2

Opening inhalation: 1 drop balsam fir

Clearing the field: 1 drop juniper berry

Soles of the feet: 1 drop ginger per foot

Along the spine/sacrum: 2 drops pine needle

Specific work: 1 drop spearmint

Closing oil: 1 drop juniper berry

. . . . . .

Deep tissue aromatherapy massage template #3

Opening inhalation: 1 drop rosemary

Clearing the field: 1 drop lime

Soles of the feet: 1 drop spearmint per foot

Along the spine/sacrum: 2 drops pine needle

Specific work: 1 drop peppermint

Closing oil: 1 drop basil

. . . . . .

Swedish massage aromatherapy template #4

Opening inhalation: 1 drop lavender

Clearing the field: 2 drops lemon

Soles of the feet: 2 drops frankincense per foot

Along the spine/sacrum: 2 drops ylang ylang

Specific work: 1 drop balsam fir

Closing oil: 1 drop lemon

. . . . . .

Swedish massage aromatherapy template #5

Opening inhalation: 2 drops tangerine

Clearing the field: 2 drops bergamot

Soles of the feet: 2 drops geranium per foot

Along the spine/sacrum: 2 drops ylang ylang or rose absolute

Specific work: 1 drop lavender

Closing oil: 1 drop bergamot

. . . . . .

Swedish massage aromatherapy template #6

Opening inhalation: 2 drops sweet orange

Clearing the field: 2 drops geranium

Soles of the feet: 2 drops ylang ylang per foot

Along the spine/sacrum: 2 drops neroli

Specific work: 1 drop lavender

Closing oil: 1 drop sweet orange

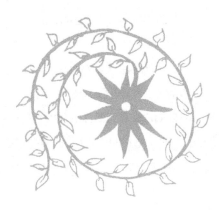

ESSENTIAL OIL & RELATED RESOURCES

Essential Oil Suppliers

Ananda Apothecary
www.anandaapothecary.com
excellent source for cacao (chocolate) essential oil and harder-to-find oils
such as palo santo, rosalina, various eucalyptus varieties, amber blends,
and CO2 extractions

Birch Hill Happenings
www.birchhillhappenings.com
private company with a vast array of essential oils and
aromatherapy supplies (bottles, pipettes, etc.);
their sweet marjoram is by far one of the loveliest and sweetest available

Starwest Botanicals
www.starwest-botanicals.com
excellent source for French green clay, dried roses and lavender, and
a good selection of essential oils; also high-quality non-irradiated bulk
herbs and spices

NOW Foods
www.nowfoods.com
high-quality, affordable, and gas chromatography-tested essential oils.
Excellent prices for 1-3 ounce bottles of best-selling NOW essential oils
can be found at Swanson Vitamins: www.swansonvitamins.com

Eden Botanicals
www.edenbotanicals.com
lovely high-quality and exotic essential oils

The Essential Oil Company
www.essentialoil.com
specializing in rare floral absolutes

Amrita Aromatherapy

http://www.amrita.net

Amrita offers a huge selection of organic, wild-crafted, and environmentally-conscious essential oils. Also a resource for hard-to-find specialty oils such as red mandarin and blue cypress.

Flora Medica

http://www.floramedica.com

excellent quality essential oils for purchase and highly-recommended certification course by a registered nurse

Green Valley Aromatherapy

www.57aromas.com

Canada-based company; selection of diffusers and nebulizers

Gritman Essential Oils

www.gritman.com

extensive variety of rare and exotic essential oils and rare macerations

Wyndmere Essential Oils

http://www.wyndmerenaturals.com

wonderful line of essential oils and products; also *highly recommended pre-diluted, affordable precious oils such as Roman chamomile, rose otto, and angelica root*

Young Living Essential Oils

www.youngliving.com

high quality therapeutic grade essential oils;
available only through distributors

doTerra

www.doterra.com

high quality therapeutic grade essential oils; available through distributors

AromaTools

www.aromatools.com

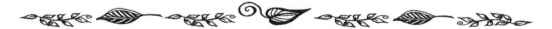

extensive variety aroma tools including bottles, containers, diffusers, nebulizers, personal care, etc.

Shaman's Dawn
www.shamansdawn.com
good source for palo santo spray

Heritage Store
www.heritagestore.com
essential oils and holistic products
based on the Edgar Cayce readings
Excellent source of rosewater

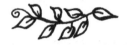

Clinical Aromatherapy and Aromatic Medicine Education

Institute of Spiritual Healing and Aromatherapy (ISHA)
www.ishaaromatherapy.com
Highly recommended 240 hour course in aromatic medicine, vibrational aromatherapy, basic essential oil composition and chemistry, and ancient spiritual healing techniques. Recognized by NAHA (The National Association of Holistic Aromatherapy) and AIA (Alliance of International Aromatherapists)

Essential Oil Resource Consultants
http://www.essentialorc.com
research and education in clinical and medical aromatherapy; distant education and courses

Flora Medica
http://www.floramedica.com

recommended certification course by a registered nurse and excellent-quality essential oils for purchase

The East West School for Herbal and Aromatic Studies
www.theida.com

Jeanne Rose Aromatherapy and All Things Herbal
www.jeannerose.net/courses.html

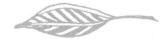

Clinical Journals and Online Resources

International Journal of Aromatherapy
http://www.ijca.net
an in-depth periodical of advanced clinical aromatherapy applications, studies, and findings

Organizations

The National Association for Holistic Aromatherapy (NAHA)
http://www.NAHA.org

RECOMMENDED AUTHORS

Barbara Brennan

Jane Buckle PhD RN

James L. Oschman

Shirley Price

Kurt Schnaubelt Ph.D.

Linda L Smith

Robert Tisserand

Valerie Ann Worwood

Gary Young, ND

BIBLIOGRAPHY

Chevallier, Andrew. Encyclopedia of Herbal Medicine. London, England: DK Publishing, 2000

Braverman, Eric R. The Edge Effect. NY, NY: Sterling Publishing Co., INC., 2004

Edwards, Victoria H. The Aromatherapy Companion. North Adams, MA: Storey Publishing, 1999

Friedman, Terry Shepherd. Freedom Through Health. Eugene, OR : Harvest Publishing, 1998

McIntyre, Anne. Flower Power. NY,NY: Henry Holt and Co., 1996

Price, Shirley. Aromatherapy for Health Professionals, 3rd Edition. London, England: Churchill Livingstone Elsevier, 2007

Ryman, Daniele. Aromatherapy. NY,NY: Bantam Books, 1991

Schnaubelt, Kurt. The Healing Intelligence of Essential Oils: The Science of Advanced Aromatherapy. Toronto, CA: Healing Arts Press, 2011

Smith, Linda L. Healing Oils, Healing Hands. HTSM Press, 2003

Tisserand, Robert. The Art of Aromatherapy. Rochester, VT: Healing Arts Press, 1978

Worwood, Valerie Ann. Aromatherapy for the Soul. Novato, CA: New World Library, 1999

Worwood, Valerie Ann. The Complete Book of Essential Oils and Aromatherapy. San Rafael, CA: New World Library 1991

Worwood, Valerie Ann. The Fragrant Mind. Novato, CA: New World Library, 1996

Young, Gary. Essential Oil Desk Reference. Essential Science Publishing, 2004

CATEGORIZED INDEX

ESSENTIAL OIL & ESSENTIAL OIL RELEVENCY INDEX

Essential Oil Profiles

Related Essential Oil References

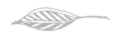

HEALTH INDEX

Acetylcholine, 43, 127, 222

Acne, 82, 83, 104, 113, 121, 126, 127, 142, 148, 150, 155, 166, 167, 169, 183, 194

A.D.D, 19

Addiction, 31, 78, 85, 111, 132, 136, 177, 222, 223, 280

ADHD, 19, 78, 91, 92, 96, 109, 142, 222

Adrenal exhaustion, 18, 116, 117, 125, 150, 151, 162

Adrenalin, 16, 17, 59, 119, 134, 193, 223

Adrenals, 17, 42, 74, 80, 84, 100, 117, 118, 122, 132, 139, 151, 162, 171, 178, 190, 223, 249, 250, 288, 289

Afternoon sluggishness, 78, 85, 112, 124, 132, 165, 170, 175, 234, 235

Age spots, 66, 67, 169

Alcoholism, 76, 77 (see also Addiction)

Allergies, seasonal, 56, 96, 113, 126, 158, 211-12

Allergy, ragweed, 96, 97, 133

Alopecia, 91, 92, 170, 174

Alzheimer's disease, 91,119, 127, 150, 151

Anemia, 137, 138

Angina, 106

Anorexia nervosa, 74, 79, 96, 105

Antibiotics, 15, 65, 150, 154

Antidepressants, 31, 39, 125, 188

Anxiety, 58, 59, 94, 100, 119, 120, 133, 146, 177, 222, 229-33

Appetite, 64, 77, 82, 88, 93, 96, 105, 109, 115, 124, 127, 130, 141, 182

Arteriosclerosis, 91, 128, 129, 137

Arthritis (see Osteoarthritis and Rheumatoid Arthritis)

Aspirin, 38, 84, 102, 175, 192, 207

Candida albicans, 64, 97, 102, 113, 121, 122, 124, 127, 137, 138, 146, 147, 157, 158, 171, 180, 183, 185

Cardiovascular system, 154

Carpal tunnel syndrome, 94, 95

Cell nutrition, 16

Cellulite, 93, 94, 103, 125, 127, 156, 181

Chemical imbalances, 96

Chemotherapy, 32, 33, 88, 89, 94, 95, 124, 125, 136, 138, 146, 147

Chicken pox, 122, 164, 165, 197

Chilblains, 124

Cholera, 86, 106, 113

Cholesterol, 89, 100, 128, 146, 147, 213

Cholinesterase, 127

Chronic fatigue syndrome, 85, 130, 178, 183, 218-20, 347

Chronic rhinitis, 99

Circulation, 16, 61, 77, 79, 84, 102, 106, 107, 124, 125, 126, 132, 137, 139, 141, 143, 152, 157, 158, 163, 164, 182, 198-99

Cirrhosis, 132

Colds (see also Flu), 28, 54, 55, 77, 79, 83, 88, 93, 104, 111, 117, 124, 132, 153, 157, 158, 162, 163, 165, 166, 170, 175, 183, 244-5, 279

Colitis, 88, 157, 158

Concentration/focus, 79, 101, 127, 129, 151, 157, 161, 222, 313

Connective tissue, 106, 107, 138, 139, 188, 189

Constipation, 64, 76, 89, 124, 152, 156, 175, 181, 216

Contraindications, 30, 32, 34, 38, 51, 56, 76, 77, 101, 116, 125, 175, 205

Coughs, 55, 57, 73, 88, 105, 118, 124, 128, 132, 143, 148, 150, 162, 163, 175, 178, 185

Cravings, 78, 84, 85, 100, 102, 109, 111, 124, 127,132, 133, 151, 223, 224, 225, 233-34

Insomnia, 18, 82, 91, 133, 144, 148, 149, 161, 171, 173, 177, 187, 188, 193, 200-1, 222, 223

Insulin, 31, 32, 94, 105, 109, 126, 133

Interferon, 33

Intestinal flora, 15,125, 137

Intoxication, 37, 39

Irregular heartbeat, 144

Irritable Bowel Syndrome, 94, 128, 157, 163, 164

Jetlag, 171

Kidney disease, 37, 85, 133

Lactation, 76, 93, 115

Lethargy, 103, 157

Leukemia, 101

Libido, 84, 90, 108, 124, 131

Limbic brain, 74, 75, 79, 85, 100

Linolenic acids, 169

Listeria, 101

Liver detoxification, (see Live health) 93

Liver health, 126, 136, 192

Low blood sugar, 32, 101, 103, 105, 109, 133, 135, 170

Low body temperature, 124

Lung congestion / lung support, (see also Coughs) 55, 81, 83, 88, 92, 141, 148, 157, 160, 178, 185, 247

Lupus, 104, 139

Luteal phase, 189

Lyme disease, 101, 102, 136, 153

Lymphatic drainage, 199

Lymphatic system, 80, 93, 107, 124, 127, 132, 137, 139, 141, 182, 199

Malaria, 80, 113

Malignancies, (see also individual Cancers) 106

Massage modalities, 16, 20, 178, 187, 198, 199, 210, 211, 225, 312-17

Massage therapists, 117, 123, 232, 312-17

Measles, 105

Medications, 11, 37, 38, 39, 102, 125, 128, 139, 188, 279, 313

Melancholy, (see also Depression), 78, 90, 96, 98, 108, 129, 130, 144, 145, 146, 148, 224

Melanoma, (see also Cancer 146)

Melatonin, 91, 92

Menopause, 18, 100, 121, 156, 158, 177, 188, 190, 191, 232, 233, 202-3

Menstrual cycle, 122, 145, 188, 230, 232, 233

Menstrual pain, 75, 94, 95, 105, 131, 143, 163, 164, 182

Miscarriage, 189, 190

Morning sickness, 88, 96

MRSA, 121, 139

Mucus membranes, 39, 41, 80, 97, 98, 154, 159, 176, 185

Multiple sclerosis, 99, 129, 161, 162, 170

Muscle injury, 24, 55, 56, 61, 117, 124

Muscle spasm, 73, 121, 157, 175, 182

Myalgic Encephalomyelitis (ME) (see Chronic Fatigue Syndrome)

Myofascial pain, 16, 60, 210-11

Nail fungus, 68, 183

Nausea, 33, 64, 75, 76, 79, 88, 89, 90, 94, 95, 103, 124, 125, 136, 158, 171, 175, 176

Nervous exhaustion, 73, 74, 88, 105, 119, 130, 140, 154, 171, 183

Nervous system, 12, 15, 16, 17, 18, 24, 27, 33, 43, 50, 58, 59, 74, 78, 79, 81, 82, 92, 94, 96, 99, 100, 109, 119, 120, 126, 133, 139, 140, 141, 148, 150, 157, 158, 161, 163, 167, 171, 173, 176, 184, 188, 189, 193, 222, 224, 249, 250, 291, 313, 314

Pet health, 18, 39, 90, 104

Petrochemicals, 51

pH balance, 18

Phlegm, 77, 83, 110, 115

Phobias, 17, 96, 101, 119, 143, 241-2

Photosensitivity, 39, 83, 139, 141, 161

Pineal, 19, 173, 190, 291

Pituitary, 119, 120, 190, 291

Pneumonia, 57, 137

Polycystic ovarian syndrome, 189

Poor memory, 78, 170, 175, 222

Post nasal drip, 110, 115

Post-traumatic stress disorder (P.T.S.D.), 129, 223, 237-9 (*Coping with Trauma blends*)

Post-workout soreness, 60, 176, 208

Pregnancy, 40, 142, 143, 173

Premature ejaculation, (see also Erectile Dysfunction) 126

Premenstrual syndrome, 85, 156, 176, 186, 188, 189

Progesterone, 100, 188, 189, 190

Prolactin, 75

Prostate, enlarged (BPH), 148, 190 (prostate support)

Pseudomonas bacteria, 153

Psoriasis, 122, 128, 129, 148, 169

Radiation treatment, 133, 134, 169, 192

Rashes, 31, 95, 122, 132, 135, 138, 148, 149

Raynaud's syndrome, (see also Circulation)124

Red blood cell production, 188, 189

Retinol, 169

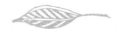

APPLICATIONS AND SYNGERGISTIC BLENDS INDEX

GENERAL INDEX

ABOUT THE AUTHOR

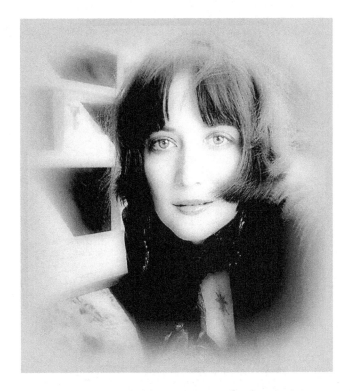

Marlaina Donato is a professional essential oil therapist specializing in clinical applications. After eleven years of independent study and use of essential oils, in 2006 she received certification from the Institute of Spiritual Healing and Aromatherapy (ISHA) led by Linda L. Smith, R.N. in Arlington, VA and certification in massage and bodywork from Applied Kinesthetic Studies in Herndon, VA.

Her interest in essential oils began after her life was altered by Chronic Fatigue Syndrome and severe Fibromyalgia at the age of 23, and due to multiple chemical sensitivities, began creating her own perfumes and body care products that her body could tolerate. It was not long until her journey led her to the deeper, life-changing health benefits of essential oils and a profound remission after eleven years of illness and near-debilitating anxiety. At the time of publication of this book, Marlaina considers herself blessed to be *living* this path of aromatic therapy for two decades. Through life challenges, health relapses and remissions, and continued self-study, she attributes her deep quality of life and sanity to essential oil therapy. Her passion is to pass on her knowledge and experience so others may also know the immeasurable wealth of this exquisite and healing art form.

Marlaina lives with her husband Joe in beautiful rural New Jersey and is the author of several books in the non-fiction and fiction genres. She is also a professional visual artist. Visit her website at: **www.marlainadonato.com**

Made in the USA
Coppell, TX
08 April 2020